Illustrated Living History Series

REVOLUTIONARY
MEDICINE
1700-1800

C. Keith Wilbur

Chelsea House Publishers

Philadelphia

Contents

Foreword

Educating the Revolutionary Physician   1
    Varied Abilities—medical schools a rarity
    Apprentice System—the preferred and practical path
    Big City Advantages—occasional lectures for the fortunate
    Anatomy—wax models and drawings more acceptable to the public than
    "Resurrectionist" activities

Quality of Care   4
Early regimental screening; four medical quacks
    Hasty Guidelines—vague Congressional regulations for the Medical Department

The Hospital   5
Medical Department positions and duties
    Director-Generals—plagued by disaster
        Dr. Benjamin Church, Dr. John Morgan, Dr. William Shippen

No Shortage on Theories   8
The Struggle to understand illness
    Revelation! Excessive or insufficient nerve stimulation caused disease!

Basic Treatments   10
    Removing Excessive Irritability
        Bloodletting technique, Blisters, Cataplasms, Formentation, Clysters
    Medications
        Anodynes, Antiarthritics, Antidysentery, Antipyretics, Emetics, Muscular spasm,
        Purgatives or Cathartics, Salivation, Sudorifics or Diaphoretics, Diuretics
    Decreased Tissue Irritability
        Anodynes, Cathartics, Clysters, Rubefacients, Stimulants, Diet

Epidemics   13
Symptoms and Treatment
    Smallpox—early inoculation of troops, technique
    Typhus—scourge of close living
    Typhoid
    Dysentery
    Diphtheria and/or Scarlet Fever
    Colds to Influenza
    Yellow Fever
    Dengue Fever
    Malaria
    Venereal Diseases
    Tory-rot

Routine Camp Ailments   17
Symptoms and treatment
    Infectious Arthritis
    Leg Sores—with bread and milk poultice recipe
    Impetigo
    Heat stroke—soldiers' drinking cups
    Drowning—resuscitation techniques, soldiers' canteens

The Army Apothecary   20
Dr. Mercer's Shop
    Medicines in short supply—collecting native medicinals
    Druggists
    Apothecaries—services offered. The first prescription. "Sovereign remedies."
        Importance of apothecary to Continental Army.
    Another first—America's pharmacopoeia
    Crude medicinals—appearance and use of raw medicines
    Signs of the times—both strange and familiar symbols
    Extracting the Active Ingredient
        Infusion, Decoction, Tincture
    Preparing Compounds
        Base, Additives, Correctives, Vehicles (electuaries, pills, ointments, liniments,
        salves, mixtures, demulcents, emollients, formentations, spirits, elixirs),
        Gas-generating apparatus

Surgery   27
Surgeons and physicians one and the same
        Directions for emergency care, Early ambulances
    Surgical equipment—regimental surgeon checklist
    Scarcity—desperate need for equipment, Medicine chest
    Principles of Healing
        Stage of inflammation, Stage of digestion
    Capital instruments—illustrated
    Notes on wounds
        Simple wounds, Puncture wounds, Gunshot wounds, Cannon ball wounds,
        Tendon wounds, For any wound—bleeding, Burns
Notes on fractures—techniques
Notes on amputations
Notes on trepanning
Further cutting remarks
        The flying hospital—emergency battle care, "Chew a bullet," Contamination cure,
        Heads or Tails? Those tell-tale wounds, The Purple Heart, Frontier surgery—
        hair-raising adventures, Teeth extraction—technique, Washington's dentures

European Medicine   41
    British and Hessians—admiration and disgust
    French—Dr. Jean Coste. Combating scurvy and smallpox. Strange hospital
        management, military pharmacopoeia

Hospitals   43
    Small house hospitals
    Big is best? Pack 'em in! Description and locations
    Big wasn't best! House of horrors with examples
    Small hospitals in favor. Dr. Tilton leads the way back to simple small structures.
        Wigwam prototype, Log hospital plan, Tents have their place
    Hospital discipline
    Corps of invalids—recycling the wounded
    Convalescent hospitals—Connecticut leads the way

An Ounce of Prevention   49
Dr. Rush an enthusiastic advocate
    Personal hygiene
        Skin, Shaving, Hair, Proper dress, Shoes
    Healthy Campsites

Tenting
Heat
Air
Bedding—by contrast, Gen. Washington's camp bed
Privies
Observations—general thoughts on camp health by Dr. Rush
A further observation—an unexpected ally—retreat
Victuals—camp cookery
Water—do's and don'ts
Spirits of '76—the joys and woes of liquid tranquilizers. Washington's liquor
   case and typical glassware

Stresses in Battle   56
The effects of excessive heat, surgery, pulmonary consumption, hardships,
homesickness, and imminent battle on the Continental soldier

Stresses on Friends and Enemy   57
Civilian reactions to the fortunes and failures of war. "Protection fever.'

Sea Surgeons   58
   Cookbook medicine for smaller vessels
   Seasickness—anatomy of the ship
   Scurvy
   Preservation of victuals—naval regulations
   Sickbay
   Advice for sea surgery
      Inventory, Ready for battle, Preparation, During action, After the engagement

The Pay Crunch   64

Revolutionary Highlights   65
   Revere Also a Dentist?
   Dr. Prescott's Ride Into History
   The Canadian Threat
   Arnold's Patriotic Leg
   Unmasking Another Traitor
   The Doctors Warren
   Signing the Declaration
   Heal Without Harm
   Apothecary Firsts
   A Valley Forge Impression
   The Perkins Tractor Cure
   Mysteries of the Mind
   The Madness of King George III
   And in Conclusion—Divided Spectacles

Certification Award   78
Paul Revere border

References

Where Illustrated Relics May Be Found

Index

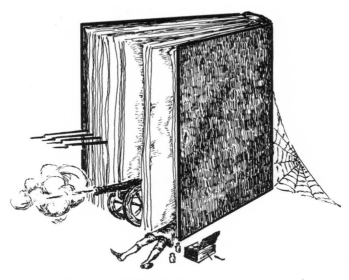

FOREWORD

There may be some exciting reading on that dusty back shelf of the medical school or hospital library! By-passed by time and the rapidity of medical progress, the ancient books still hold past victories over disease, trial-and-error remedies, and surgical challenges.

But what of the patient who asks if a flaxseed poultice could relieve a stitch or if he should stuff a cold and starve a fever (or is it the other way around?!). Does grandmother's borax really make an effective mouthwash? Should Epsom salts be used to soak that sore foot, and are sulfur baths still useful for impetigo? And "Why did you doctors take to bleeding in the old days?" The old medical arts seem better remembered by the patient rather than his physician.

Some of the answers are in the following pages. There are no self-improvement quizzes to take~ no postgraduate exams to worry through. It's a short retroscopic view of medicine two centuries ago, its involvement in the Revolutionary War, and how our earlier physicians met the staggering medical crisis in Washington's army.

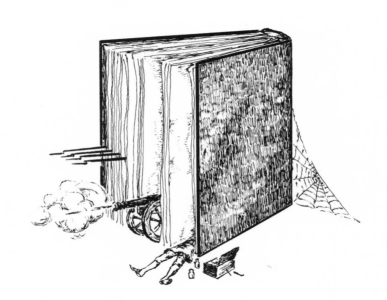

EDUCATING THE REVOLUTIONARY PHYSICIAN

VARIED ABILITIES ~ The momentum of Lexington and Concord had carried the colonial militia to British-occupied Boston Town. It seemed little more than an armed rabble, poorly trained and ill-equipped to face the strongest military power of the Eighteenth Century. Each regiment in this civilian army had brought its own physician. Medical and surgical treatment by these men - known as regimental surgeons - seemed even less likely of success than that of their military brothers. They were hometown doctors of varied ability, and needed only the approval of the regimental commander and a rubber stamp from the colonial legislature before receiving their commissions.

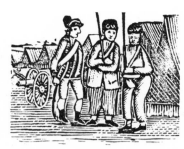

A BRITISH SATIRE ON THE REBEL CAMPS NEAR BOSTON.

These regimental surgeons were part of the 3500 practicing physicians in the colonies in 1775. Of these, less than 300 had received a medical degree. Only a handful had graduated from the ten-year-old Philadelphia Medical College. The remainder, mainly from the middle and southern colonies, attended the European medical schools. Admission requirements included a knowledge of the classics and a husky bank roll. By the time the graduating thesis had been written in Latin, the student had been exposed to all the latest theories that Edinburgh, London, or the Continent had to offer. Theories aplenty - but the fledgling M.D.'s returned to America without having seen a patient!

APPRENTICE SYSTEM ~ The bulk of the practicing physicians in the colonies - including all of the independent New Englanders - were apprentice-trained. Some had undergraduate degrees, while others were no more than fifteen years old when starting their medical careers. Dr. Benjamin Rush noted that the only prerequisite for a "doctor's boy" was the ability to stand the sight of blood! His teacher was likely a prominent physician-surgeon, well qualified to guide the student through the maze of anatomy, osteology, the compounding of medicine, surgery, and the writings of Hippocrates. Toward the end of the three-to-six year apprenticeship, the doctor's boy was doing his own bloodletting, tooth-pulling, dressing wounds and some minor surgery. His certificate of proficiency gave the same practicing privileges as a medical school degree.

THESE May Inform all Whom it might Concern That Mr. John Kaighin of Hatfield in the Province of West New Jersey, hath Lived with me (here under named) a considerable time, as a Disciple, to Learn the Arts & Mysteries of Chymistry, Physick, & the Astral Sciences, whereby to make a more perfect Discovery of the Hidden causes of More Occult & uncommon Diseases, not so easily to be discovered by the Vulgar Practice. In all which he has been very Diligent & Studious, as well as in the Administeration of the Medecines, & in the Various Cases; wherein his Judgment may be safely depended upon, all things, so far as he follows my Instructions. And Hope he may in all things answer the Confidence that may be reposed in him.
Germantown Febr: 30. 1738.
C. Witt.

CERTIFICATE OF PROFICIENCY.

This practical bedside approach persisted well into our Twentieth Century. It had other advantages for any young, impressionable student living under the same roof as his preceptor. The doctor became a father figure - an ideal to follow. Since physicians have always been an independent lot, American freedom was a popular subject. When the conflict with England became reality, the medical profession gave outstanding service to their country as healers, law-makers and military leaders.

An apprenticeship was not without its heavy moments under hard taskmasters. Dr. John Redman, who apprenticed such outstanding Revolutionary war doctors as Rush, Morgan and Shippen, was hard used by a physician of "morose and churlish temper." He was pressed into service as a coachman, messenger boy, prescription clerk and nurse. When Rush studied under Dr. Redman he likewise repaid his excellent teacher by taking charge of the doctor's book and accounts. He was absent from his duties but eleven days during his five-year apprenticeship.

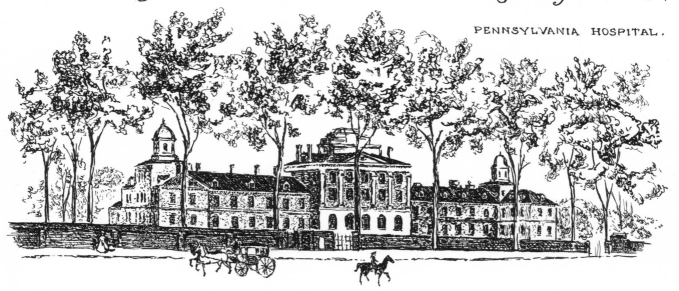

DR. JOHN REDMAN (1722-1808) FROM A CONTEMPORARY CARTOON.

BIG CITY ADVANTAGES ~ Apprentices in the larger cities - Philadelphia - Boston - New York - had prospects of sitting in on medical lectures. The first and best of such systematic efforts was centered in Philadelphia. In November of 1762, Dr. Shippen began his series on anatomy, diseases, cures, surgical procedures, methods of bandaging and "a few plain directions on midwifery." It was a whirlwind tour through the fine points of Eighteenth Century medicine. When the osteology course ended in February of 1763, the Philadelphia Gazette mentioned "...Osteology - the most dry, though the most necessary part of anatomy." Twentieth Century medical students still know the meaning of "dry as a bone"!

PENNSYLVANIA HOSPITAL.

In that same city, the Pennsylvania Hospital was considered the ultimate in medical care in the Colonies. Doctors brought their "boys" on round for firsthand observation. By 1773 the hospital began its own apprentice system. After five years, the successful candidate was awarded a certificate and a suit of "cloathes."

ANATOMY ~ Hermanus Carroll did not die in vain in 1750. Although executed for murder in New York City, his mortal remains made medical history at the first dissection for medical students. There were others - most to remain forever nameless - who were raised from the grave by the "Resurrectionists." Teachers and students alike pursued this nocturnal activity, so great was the need for anatomical knowledge. Deceased indigents and paupers were the best bets - there were few relatives to ask questions.

But there **were** questions. Mobs gathered in protest. Dr. Shippen's Philadelphia dissection room windows were smashed and the doctor ran for his life on several occasions. His home was attacked and his carriage ventilated with shot. Shippen tried to quiet the uproar with several newspaper notices. He assured the locals that private burying grounds were never disturbed, and that only suicides and those publicly executed were selected as subjects—except "now and then one from the Potter's Field."

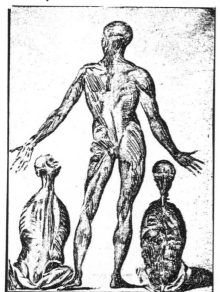

ONE OF THE CRAYON ANATOMICAL DRAWINGS USED BY DR. SHIPPEN

Lacking anatomical material, large drawings were substituted. One year before Lexington and Concord, Dr. Abraham Chovet was using remarkable wax molds of the body, as well as injected and preserved anatomical preparations. His announcements in 1774-75 read:

"As the course cannot be attended with the disagreeable sight or smell of recent disease and putrid carcasses, which often disgust even the students in Physick, as well as the curious, otherwise inclined to this useful and sublime part of natural philosophy, it is hoped this understanding will meet with suitable encouragement."

John Adams was apparently one of the "curious," and evidently gave "suitable encouragement." His diary on October 14, 1774 noted:

"Went in the morning to see Dr. Chovet, and his skeletons and wax works—most admirable, exquisite representations of the whole animal economy. Four complete skeletons, a leg with all the nerves, veins, and arteries injected with wax, two complete bodies in wax, full grown; waxen representations of all the muscles, tendons &c., of the head, brain, heart, lungs, liver, stomach &c. This exhibition is much more exquisite than that of Dr. Shippen at the hospital."

Early in the Revolution, the body of a soldier was removed from its grave—and the coffin left open. Dr. Thacher wrote of the great upsurge of grief and resentment among the "populace. The "Resurrectionists" went undiscovered, but Washington was so moved by the incident that he strictly prohibited such practice in the future. However, when Dr. John Warren was in charge of the Continental Army hospital at Boston, there was an abundance of unclaimed dead. Dissections were frequent during his lectures to those Harvard students planning to study medicine.

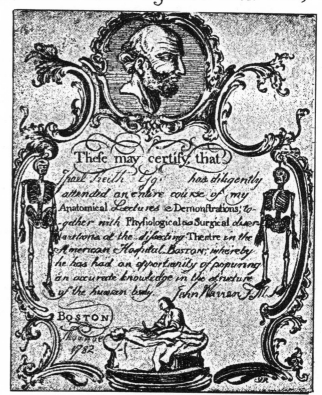

CERTIFICATE OF ATTENDANCE FOR DR. WARREN'S LECTURES, 1782. ENGRAVED BY REVERE.

QUALITY OF CARE

Smith's "History of New York," written shortly after the Revolution, summed up the lack of quality medical standards. "Few physicians amongst us are eminent for their skill. Quacks abound and too many have recommended themselves to a full and profitable practice and substance. Any man at his pleasure sets up for physician, apothecary, or chirurgeon. No candidates are examined or licensed. In Connecticut where a movement was instituted to require physicians to pass an examination to practice, the assembly decided in favor of the irregulars and against any monopoly in the practice of medicine."

The apprentice system is not ancient history. Indeed, it has persisted into our present century. Even after American medical schools had taken over the bulk of the physicians' education, there were no qualification standards until as late as 1910.

Around besieged Boston, the contrast in medical care became painfully obvious. Only Massachusetts, with the war in her own front yard, made haste to require examinations of her regimental surgeons. Dr. James Thacher, in his "Military Journal," described his close and severe examination. Two Massachusetts Commission physicians pounded away at sixteen medical militia appointees. After four hours of a concentrated quiz on anatomy, physiology, surgery and medicine, six were rejected as unqualified. The remainder, including Thacher, were accepted after promising the "faithful discharge of duty and the humane treatment of any soldier who may have the misfortune to require my assistance."

The doctor continued: "But it was on another occasion, as I am told, that a candidate under examination was agitated into a state of perspiration, and being required to describe the mode of treatment in rheumatism, among other remedies he would promote a sweat, and being asked how he would effect this with his patient, after some hesitation he replied, 'I would have him examined by a medical committee.'"

CAPᵀ SAMUEL PHILLIPS' EYE STONE. SUPERSTITION HAD IT THAT FOREIGN OBJECTS IN THE EYE COULD BE REMOVED BY THE MAGICAL POWERS OF CERTAIN STONES.

HASTY GUIDELINES

~ When Washington took command of his heterogeneous army of militiamen and volunteers around Boston's periphery, he was as troubled about the care of the sick and wounded as were the Massachusetts lawmakers. He needled Congress into initial action by writing that "... the lives of both officers and men were so much dependent on a due regulation of this medical department." The Commander-in-Chief had no intention of committing his newly organized Continental Army to battle without proper medical backup.

Congressional thinking approved of both a civilian and professional army, for this was in the spirit of democratic checks and balances. The militia and their regimental surgeons would continue their duties of home defense ~ and to bolster the army's efforts when called upon. And usually the militia **were** necessary to fill the Continental lines. Good will and cooperation between the two, with a reasonable set of guidelines to follow, could only strengthen America's bid for freedom. Unfortunately, the medical men of both bodies squabbled like fishwives until congressional regulations became more clearly defined.

THE HOSPITAL

On July 25, 1775 - the smoke from Breeds and Bunker Hill had hardly cleared - Congress made the Continental Army medical corps a reality. In the language of the times, it was called the "Hospital" - not to be confused with a building housing the sick. A Director-General and Chief Physician was given the awesome responsibility of appointing four qualified surgeons and an apothecary for an army of twenty thousand soldiers. He must oversee the twenty surgeons' mates, a matron, one nurse for every ten patients, a clerk to keep accounts and two storekeepers that received and distributed supplies. He must "...furnish medicines, bedding, and all other necessities, pay for the same, superintend the whole, and make his report to, and receive orders from the Commander-in-Chief."

The British Army medical system was well known to the colonials from the old French and Indian War days. It had merit, for the medical administration was entirely separate from that of purveyor and the securing of supplies. But Congress was in no mood to follow anything that was British - particularly after the traitorous actions of its first Director-General. The chaos created by this double responsibility lost more than one campaign for Washington.

DIRECTOR-GENERALS ~

At any rate, the first three of the four Director-Generals of the "Hospital" left a trail of disaster behind them. Of these well-qualified and capable physicians, one turned traitor, the second was humiliated and disposed of by Regimental pressure, and the third became a victim of his own ambition and dishonesty.

Dr. Benjamin Church - July 27, 1775 to October 3, 1775. This well-educated and popular Boston physician, known as a "staunch patriot," was actually a spy. A general court-martial, presided over by Washington himself, found his first Director-General guilty of sending coded messages to the British. After a year in prison, he was allowed to go to the West Indies. The sea claimed the traitor when all hands were lost on the voyage.

Dr. John Morgan ~ October 17, 1775 to January 9, 1777. This Philadelphian was a gifted physician and teacher, the first medical professor at the College of Philadelphia, and blessed with ideals and patriotism beyond reproach. With characteristic energy, he worked to bring efficiency and discipline to the Hospital of the Continental Army. Unfortunately, he lacked diplomacy and was an authoritarian - qualities much too close to the aristocratic and overbearing manners of the stereotyped Tory.

For starters, Congress had provided no rules or guidelines. Therefore Morgan urged that regimental surgeons be quality controlled by being screened and appointed by his office. Failing this, he tried to bring the independent and often cantankerous regimental surgeons under Hospital regulations. No response. He then insisted that the regimental hospitals send their severely ill and wounded militiamen to the Continental Hospital staff

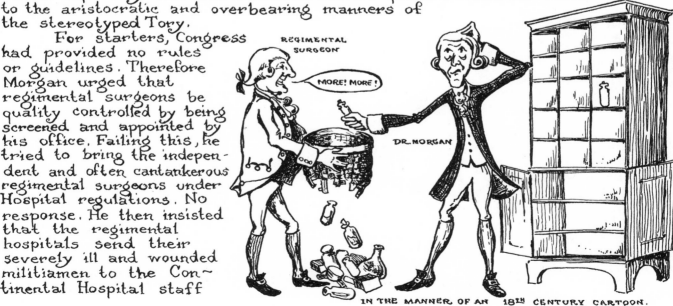

REGIMENTAL SURGEON

MORE! MORE!

DR. MORGAN

IN THE MANNER OF AN 18TH CENTURY CARTOON.

for care. The regimental surgeons, finding themselves little more than first aid stations, rebelled by sending along the contagious patients – and any surplus that had accumulated. Their commanders fired off critical letters to Congress. Morgan fired a few volleys himself when he exploded to Congress that they were "men of the same mean, sordid, groveling disposition" as their militia, who in turn were peppered with "malingerers, public extortioners and cowards."

But it was probably Morgan's efforts as a glorified quartermaster that caused the greatest uproar. In addition to the frustrating business of trying to provide the army with quality medical care, he managed to seek out the meager supplies of medicines for the Hospital. The regimental surgeons, as allowed by Congress, felt free to draw all manner of provisions. The Director-General threw up his hands and cried, "We are now scarcely any thing more than collectors and retailers to the Regimental Surgeons and Mates." One surgeon in Cambridge drew out one hundred gallons of rum and proportional amounts of wine, loaf and brown sugar and molasses; "...and to shew the extreme necessity, one pint of oatmeal was added to the list, being for one regiment only; all within the space of about six weeks ....."

DIRECTOR-GENERAL JOHN MORGAN.

Washington appreciated and sympathized with his Director-General's dilemma. Unless the British medical system and some hard and fast regulations came from Congress, complete chaos would be the lot of Continental and militia medicine. Meanwhile the General made it clear as to just who were the troublemakers.

"The regimental surgeons I am speaking of," he wrote Congress in September of 1776, "many of whom are very great rascals, contenancing the men to sham complaints to exempt them from duty, and often receiving bribes to certify indispositions with a view to procure discharges and furloughs." Further, "The regimental surgeons are aiming, I am pursuaded, to break up the General Hospital, and have in numberless instances drawn from medicines, stores, etc., in the most profane and extravagant manner for private purposes."

GENERAL WASHINGTON REVIEWING TROOPS. FROM 1795 OIL PAINTING.

July, 1776 – it was a momentous month with bonfires, parades, bells and cannon salutes announcing the Declaration of Independence. The British moved to dampen the festivities by an invasion of Long Island and New York. And Dr. Morgan took solid steps to bring some well-defined regulations to the civilian and Continental medical department. At a joint meeting, it was resolved that the regiments would continue their own hospitals and to make daily reports to their commanding officers. Severely ill militiamen would be sent to the General Hospital for the same care as the Continental soldiers – provided none had "infections, putrid or malignant" diseases that might spread to others. Full information would accompany the new admissions. The regimental surgeons would draw necessities for their medical chest from the Hospital, but other supplies would come from the Regimental Quartermaster. And one further regulation - a guard was to be posted at each regimental hospital to maintain discipline, preventing patients from wandering about and to stop unauthorized visitors. The British system was gradually becoming a part of American medicine.

But Dr. John Morgan's considerable abilities were soon lost to the young nation. Congress reacted to the crush of criticism and discharged him without explanation. The former Director-General petitioned for a public hearing to save the only thing left - his good name. Finally, on June 12, 1779, Congress finally admitted that he was guiltless of wrongdoing.

Ten years later, it was Dr. Benjamin Rush who discovered his old friend's body in a small hovel. Broken and lonely, he had died amidst a profusion of medical books and papers. Rush's diary was something of an epitaph. "What a change from his former rank and prospects in Life! The man who once filled half the world with his name, had now scarcely friends enough to bury him."

Dr. William Shippen. April 11, 1777 ~ January 3, 1781. This Philadelphia physician was well-known for giving the first systematic medical courses in the Colonies, and three years later as Professor of Anatomy at the College of Philadelphia. When the first medical school was established shortly thereafter, he fancied himself snubbed by Dr. Morgan. This slight festered into an obsession to place his former friend as Director-General - despite being made director of the New Jersey Flying Camp field hospital by Morgan.

DIRECTOR-GENERAL WILLIAM SHIPPEN.

Shippen had his foot in the door. With the help of Dr. John Cochran, Congress was presented with a plan that progressed further toward the British system. Military districts were proposed for the Eastern, Northern, Middle and Southern theaters, with medical officers to oversee their proper function. Congress, sick of the constant wrangles that marked Dr. Morgan's administration, looked on Shippen as their fair-haired boy. He further strengthened his hand by falsifying the Flying Camp records to appear more efficient than Morgan. And his ambitions were certainly not hindered by having two brothers-in-law in Congress.

Dr. Shippen - or rather now Director-General Shippen - faced the two darkest years of the Revolution. There were few funds and fewer supplies. For these the new Director-General could not be blamed. At least half the army was moldering in the General Hospital. The crowding of the sick spread the communicable diseases like wildfire. The mortality was unbelievable. Shippen, meanwhile, paid scant attention to sanitation and crowding in the Hospital department. He apparently had other interests, for in March of 1780 he was brought to trial on charges of "Scandalous and infamous practices such are unbecoming the Character of an Officer & Gentleman" - including speculation in the sale of Hospital stores. Although acquitted by a single vote, Shippen prudently resigned his commission shortly thereafter.

Meanwhile, the Continental Congress had taken a firmer hand in the army's medical affairs. Reorganization included the Act of October 6, 1780, whereby the Director-General was given the rank of Brigadier-General. He was forever separated from the chores of purveyor, now under the Chief Physician who ranked as a Colonel. When Dr. John Cochran became the fourth Director-General, the Hospital was at last on an efficient course.

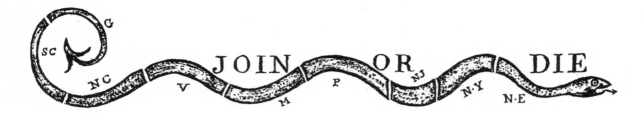

NO SHORTAGE ON THEORIES

The Eighteenth Century medical students and physicians were frequently confounded by the causes of illness. Bacteriology, pathology, biochemistry and quantitative physiology were much in the future. Meanwhile, the less known of an illness, the more the medicines prescribed. Today's physicians find it so when treating the mysteries of cancer, viral infections, the rheumatic syndromes, hypertension, alcoholism and schizophrenia.

The old Grecian theories of humors had been too comfortable to discard. The bodily fluids - blood, phlegm, black bile and yellow bile - must remain in balance for good health. An excess or deficiency of any or all resulted in disease. Bleeding, purging or sweating relieved the excess, while rest, diets and medicinals made up any defect.

Advances in physics and chemistry in the Seventeenth Century substituted acidity, alkalinity, saltiness, tension and relaxation for the old humors. It wasn't all that revolutionary, and treatment continued along the old lines. Many of the older regimental surgeons framed their practice on just such principles.

It was Thomas Sydenham (1624-1684) who lashed out at such unproven speculations. His advice was simple. Physicians should get off their backsides and get back to the bedside! Observe the patient closely, and by firsthand experience help "...nature to throw off the morbific matter." Forget the powerful R_x that did more harm than good.

Closer observation of disease encouraged experimentation. The mid-Eighteenth Century medical world was electrified when it was discovered that muscular tissue contracted when its nerves were stimulated!

PIERRE LYONET MADE THIS MICROSCOPE IN PARIS BETWEEN 1742 AND 1750.

THIS WAS THE FIRST INSTRUMENT ESPECIALLY MADE FOR MICRODISSECTION.

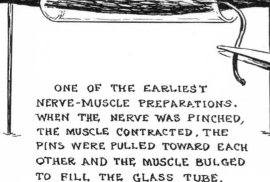

ONE OF THE EARLIEST NERVE-MUSCLE PREPARATIONS. WHEN THE NERVE WAS PINCHED, THE MUSCLE CONTRACTED, THE PINS WERE PULLED TOWARD EACH OTHER AND THE MUSCLE BULGED TO FILL THE GLASS TUBE.

ARMED FORCES INSTITUTE OF PATHOLOGY (ABOVE)

A solid physiological fact at last! The theorists were quick to turn fact into fancy. Famous physicians and lecturers in the European medical centers - particularly Edinburgh - were off and running. Dr. William Cullen taught that nerve irritation could alter the body fluids to cause illness. As a bonus, he devised a massive and complex classification of diseases. Since their causes were unknown, each combination of symptoms became a different disease. By adding up a soldier's fever, rash, aches, pains and whatnot, one could match the symptoms to the text and come up with a diagnosis.

The Scotch physician, John Brown, was not to be outdone. His Brunonian system rebelled against Cullen's hodgepodge classification, and a simple "unity" theory came into being. Good health depended upon a proper balance of nerve stimulation to muscle and blood vessel response. It seemed obvious that excessive stimulation gave muscle spasm and then on to disease. Too little stimulation gave weakness or atony. It was a satisfying bit of reasoning, for it wrapped all illnesses into a tidy package. American students hurried the new gospel back from Europe and were ready for the unsuspecting soldiers when the Revolutionary War broke out.

Actually, the ancient Greeks would have been right at home with the current treatments. Those suffering from excessive nerve stimulation (for example, fever) could be cured by the good old bleeding, purging, alcohol and low diet. Also, one might compete with the stimuli by local irritants via skin blistering, oral mercury and medicinals via mouth or rectum. Debility called for a build-up of nervous energy by restorative drugs and drinks. If "stuff a cold and starve a fever" has an unreasonable but familiar ring to it, it has been thought so for the past two hundred years.

Since theories had solved all the diagnostic problems for the moment, the Revolutionary era physician felt free to ignore Dr. Sydenham's advice. Temperatures and pulses were rarely taken, even though they were measured by Galileo a century and a half before. Blood pressures were first recorded in 1733, but slipped from the mind for one hundred and fifty more years before the sphygmomanometer was invented. A Vienna physician showed the importance of chest percussion in 1761, but the technique was not rediscovered until well after the rebellion. The Revolutionary soldier had an enemy he had not counted upon - symptomatic treatment by his physician.

LAENNEC'S FIRST STETHOSCOPE IN 1816 WAS A TIGHTLY ROLLED LENGTH OF PAPER. (LEFT)

AND ALSO TOO LATE FOR THE REVOLUTION WAS HIS THREE-PIECE WOODEN TUBE WITH A CENTRAL BORE AND DETACHABLE CHEST PIECE. (ABOVE) 1816 - 1819

BASIC TREATMENTS

Take the average healthy Continental soldier with a proper balance between nerve stimuli and the excitability of his body's tissues. Suddenly he is exposed to an exciting cause. Externally, it could be such as bad air (mal-aria), spoiled food or tainted drink, exposure to cold after excessive heat, wounds, drunkenness, or even the grating of a knife on a pewter plate. Internal causes might include any emotion or "passion." Once such stimuli irritated the nerves, spasm of the blood vessels and muscles would follow. The patient became hot and developed a rapid pulse. Tightened muscles began aching. He was obviously diseased. The army physician must set about to counter this excessive excitability.

REMOVING EXCESSIVE IRRITABILITY

1. BLOODLETTING ~ To remove excesses from the blood by depletion, bleeding was enthusiastic. Dr. Rush didn't hesitate to remove a quart of blood every forty-eight hours. (Unfortunately, it was thought the body contained twelve and not the actual six quarts of blood.) George Washington died of his infected throat ~ with the help of his physician ~ after nine pints were taken in twenty-four hours!

Procedure ~

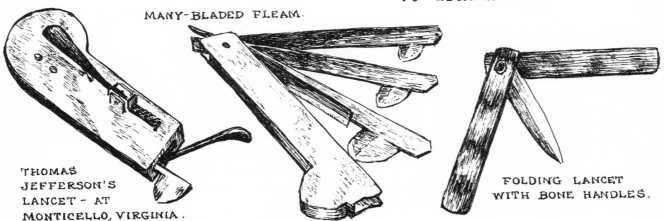

PLACE PATIENT'S HAND IN HOT WATER TO SWELL VEINS.

TIE TAPE AT THE PULSE. PATIENT OPENS HAND TWO OR THREE TIMES TO CAUSE FURTHER SWELLING.

HOLD PATIENT'S HAND BY THE FINGERS AND STRETCH. PIERCE THE VEIN LONGITUDINALLY.

FINALLY, DIP HAND IN HOT WATER TO MAKE THE BLOOD FLOW FREELY. LOOSEN TAPE TO ALLOW IMPURE BLOOD TO ESCAPE.

MANY-BLADED FLEAM.

THOMAS JEFFERSON'S LANCET ~ AT MONTICELLO, VIRGINIA.

FOLDING LANCET WITH BONE HANDLES.

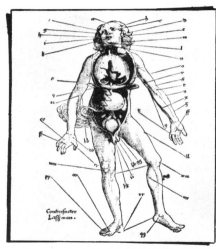

BLOODLETTING CHART BY GERMAN
JOHANNES WECHTLIN, 1540. THERE WAS NO
LACK OF SITES FOR VENESECTION!

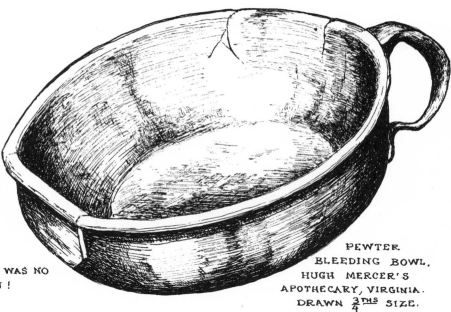

PEWTER
BLEEDING BOWL.
HUGH MERCER'S
APOTHECARY, VIRGINIA.
DRAWN $\frac{3}{4}$THS SIZE.

2. BLISTERS ~ A counterirritant to compete with tissue excitability elsewhere. Plasters were prepared by dipping flannel in caustics such as cantharides (the mash of Spanish fly ~ a green blister beetle), or by spreading the irritant on linen or leather. These were applied to the skin, and did indeed raise blisters.

3. CATAPLASMS ~ Otherwise known as poultices, to relieve pain, swelling or the discharge of pus. A hot paste of wheat bran or flaxseed was applied to the skin, then covered with flannel.

4. FORMENTATION ~ Applications of hot, moist substances to ease pain, such as flannel with hot water.

5. CLYSTERS ~ Rectal administration of medications when the oral route was more difficult.

DRAWN $\frac{3}{4}$THS SIZE.

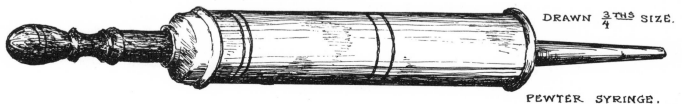

PEWTER SYRINGE.

MEDICATIONS
Since treatment was symptomatic, the Continental physician thought along the following lines:

1. ANODYNES ~ Only for lessening pain and not useful for removing the symptoms of excitability or inflammation. ℞ Opium (called Extractum Thebaicum) and Laudanum, composed of opium and Saffron, extracted with Canary wine.

2. ANTIARTHRITICS ~ ℞ Epsom salt soaks or the "Bark" (Peruvian Bark or Chinchona), containing quinine for ague.

3. ANTIDYSENTERY ~ ℞ Pul. Ipecac (pulverized Brazil Root),

11

blackberry wine and Elix. Asthmat. (elixir asthmaticum) composed of opium, honey, licorice, benzoic acid, camphor, oil of anise, potassium carbonate and alcohol. The latter is known today as *paragoric~from the Greek "Paragorican" meaning soothing. Warm baths and vomits were also used.

4. ANTIPYRETICS~
Also called Febrifuges, to prevent or reduce fever. Emetics were used to check a fever in its early stages before the patient was confined to bed. Then, "the Bark" was the popular treatment for general or malignant fevers, along with laxatives or clysters, cold baths and vomits.

5. EMETICS~
Produced vomiting. Popular for bilious attacks, dysentery, jaundice and digestive problems (to remove the irritant causing excitability) as well as for ingestion of bad water, tainted meat, fish, bread or fruits. R Tartar emetic, *ipecac, or warm water and honey until vomitus became clear.

GLASS MEDICINE BOTTLES.

CLAY MEDICINE BOTTLE.

6. MUSCULAR SPASM~
To relax, R Opium, wine (quarts or even gallons daily), ardent spirits, "the Bark," oil of amber.

7. PURGATIVES OR CATHARTICS~
Laxatives were felt to rid excessive intestinal irritation or to set up a counterirritation for excesses elsewhere. R Glauber's Salts, Plummer's Pills, ipecac, jalap, calomel, saline, rhubarb, and castor oil. Epsom salts (magnesium sulfate) was named after the famous English watering place and health spa where the waters contained magnesium sulfate.

8. SALIVATION~
Mercury in oil, held in the mouth, stimulated saliva as well as creating a counter intestinal irritant.

9. SUDORIFICS OR DIAPHORETICS~
Produces perspiration. Sweat baths were used from the early Indian days for this purpose. Felt useful after intestinal symptoms were controlled. R Camphor, Dover's Powder (opium and ipecac) and rhubarb.

10. DIURETICS~
For dropsy (edema) to increase the urine flow. It was thought that any illness would have a characteristic urine. R Milk for mild diuresis and a good diluting agent for diuretic extracts of dandelions, juniper berries or lemon juice.

WOODEN PILL BOX.

It was considered proper to use those old favorites of bloodletting, purging and blistering with any or all of the above. A low diet of thin, diluting drinks was recommended - for example, barley water, flaxseed tea, and watery gruel. Exposing the body to cool water and air also countered the fever.

TORTOISE SHELL TWEEZERS.

DECREASED TISSUE IRRITABILITY

Occasionally, nerve stimulation could exhaust the body's tissues. Weakness, atony, and general debility resulted. To build up the nervous energy one must give:

ANODYNES ~ In large doses, were felt to excite and not relax.

CATHARTICS ~ Scouring the intestine orally, or

CLYSTERS ~ A soft, soothing enema, for daily bowel movements were considered important.

RUBEFACIENTS ~ Substances to irritate and redden the skin.

STIMULANTS ~ ℞ Anise, pepper, cinnamon, cloves, dill, sage, ginger, horseradish, nutmeg, horehound, lavender, marjoram and spearmint.

DIET ~ Nourishing broths. Liquor also was given to dilate blood vessels.

EPIDEMICS

Dr. Benjamin Rush, in his "Travels Through Life," told of offending an American officer who expressed fear of dying of some camp disease. "To die of a bullet," he said, "was the natural death of a soldier." Since six of every seven deaths were due to such camp "distempers," the officer's fears were well founded. Whenever great numbers of troops from all parts of the Colonies came together, communicable diseases would be hard behind.

SMALLPOX ~ Was considered the principle disease of that century ~ and the only one with a proven prophylaxis. The British evacuation of Boston in March of 1776 left behind pockets of the illness. Hannah Winthrop wrote her friend Mercy Warren that "Men Women and Children eagerly crowding to inoculate is I think as modish as running away from the Troops of a barbarous George was the last year." The militia who decimated the redcoat ranks at Breed's Hill would hardly agree, but were ready and willing to line up with the Bostonians for their inoculations.

General Washington went his troops one better. Because his wife was a frequent visitor to the camps, he saw to it that she was inoculated in Philadelphia. Later, during the hard wintering at Morristown, he ordered all soldiers and nearby civilians to be pox-proofed. And early in 1777, all remaining troops were so treated. All new arrivals were inoculated at Philadelphia while awaiting their arms, accoutrements and clothing. Only one in a thousand failed to recover from the procedure.

A healthy donor supplied clear serum from an early vesicle. The advanced, contaminated pustules were avoided. The pock was opened with a toothpick (the patient might panic at the sight of a lancet), pressed and the matter scooped up in a quill. The serum was then introduced into the arm of the recipient through a small

BENJAMIN RUSH ~ AN OUTSTANDING PHYSICIAN OF THIS PERIOD.

scratch or puncture. Recovery followed
exposure to cold air, drinking cold water
and a dose of mercurial purgatives. It was
a tolerable prophylactic measure until
the cowpox vaccine was discovered in
England in 1798. Two years later
America was using this virus.

SIDE PRESSURE EXPRESSED THE SERUM INTO A QUILL.

TYPHUS (Hospital Fever or Jail Fever) It was known that this
contagion was transferred from the hospital to the camps by blankets
or clothes. It certainly became rampant where many troops from different
areas assembled. Lack of cleanliness fed the disease,
as did poor diet, excessive fatigue and use of linen
instead of woolen clothes in the summer. (Heavier
clothing apparently discouraged the hungry louse.)
Drunken patients, convalescents and black soldiers
were thought particularly susceptible. Astute Dr.
Rush questioned lice as a cause, well before the
discovery that rickettsia were actually spread
the bite of the body louse.
    This fearsome disease crawled among the
closely packed hospital patients to claim countless
lives. The early symptoms were innocent enough – chills
and fever, tongue covered with a yellowish green crust,
some listlessness and headache. Trembling of the hands
followed, some loss of hearing and sight, and a feeble
pulse. Lastly, the telltale petechiae – irregular purplish
spots, peeling skin and falling hair – and very possibly death.
    Emetics were considered helpful to check the fever in the
forming state. Thereafter, the treatment followed the well-worn path
of any such "excessive stimulation" diseases.

TYPHOID (Malignant Bilious Fever) was considered the same
disease as Typhus. Unnoticed differences were diarrhea and rose-colored
spots on the chest and abdomen – and the bacterial etiology, spread from
contaminated excrement on food, clothing or bedding.

DYSENTERY (Diarrhea or Flux) Causes included drinking stagnate
or marsh water, tainted food, cold air or sleeping in wet clothing. With
the fever came abdominal cramps and frequent stools of blood, pus
and mucus. Any fool could make the diagnosis, but the bacterial etiology
of typhoid was well beyond Revolutionary thought.

DIPHTHERIA AND/OR SCARLET FEVER Although of different
bacterial etiologies, these two diseases were considered the same. They
were lumped under such exotic terms as Throat Distemper, Angina
Suffocativa, Bladder In The Throat, Cynanche Trachealis, Angina
Maligna, Epidemical Eruptive Miliary Fever and Angina Ulcusculosa.
The cause was thought to be "from some Affection of the Air, and
not from any personal Infection receiv'd from the Sick, or goods
in their neighborhood." Hallmarks were the swollen white-flecked
throat, profound weakness, and the tough slime that ultimately
suffocated many patients.
    ℞ The usual bleeding followed all such "excessive stimulation"

diseases, as noted from George Washington's last hours on earth. But frequently, the treatment for this disease had a different twist. The preferred incision was under the tongue. Alum dissolved in honey and sharp vinegar served as a gargle. And there were decoctions to drink, the favorite going by the unlikely name of Devil's Bitt.

COLDS TO INFLUENZA (Tussis Epidemica, Catarrh) Etiology
included close contacts, corrupt air from animal droppings, perspiration, stale clothes and unturned bedsheets, books long shut in closed rooms, and "full living" without exercise. For eight to ten days the familiar "running at the nose," chills and fever, head pains and a troublesome cough caused their misery. The fortunate ended the viral bout with profuse sweating. Eighteenth Century medical books also noted complicating symptoms typical of bacterial pneumonitis.

YELLOW FEVER—
(The Great Sickness, The American Plague, Barbadoes Distemper, or Bilious Plague)
Jaundice gave its color— but infectious hepatitis, dengue and malaria could give the same red blood cell destruction. The undiscovered culprit was the virus-infected Aedes Aegypti. Unless carried by winds, the mosquito wasn't much of a traveller. In Rush's day, one such epidemic was confined to a single Philadelphia street. It was known, quite understandably, as Front Street Fever. The larvae, brought from the Indies in cargo ships, flourished in local rain barrels and stagnant puddles.

AEDES AEGYPTI
8-12 DAYS AFTER
BITE, SYMPTOMS APPEAR.
ONE ATTACK GAVE IMMUNITY.
MANY BLACK SOLDIERS HAD CHILD-
HOOD EXPOSURE AND WERE UNAFFECTED.

Seaports and southern camps were often plagued with violent fevers, head and back pain, and the "rigors". Vomiting, eyes "like two balls of fire," and a yellowish tinting of the skin brought the patient into the critical third to the fifth day. Prognosis was poor if he then presented with an excessive temperature, cold extremities, and burning around the region of the liver. However, the appearance of a general rash "proved salutary," according to Dr. Rush's account of the great Philadelphia epidemic of 1762.

Vinegar played an important part in prophylaxis. A bowl of the liquid in the hospital ward and "a hot iron sometimes put therein" perhaps discouraged the mosquito by its fumes. The visiting physician dipped his hands into the container before taking the pulse, and likely rubbed vinegar on his face as well. Tobacco, held in the mouth, prevented swallowing one's saliva, and it was not uncommon to see women and children about with cigars in their mouths at epidemic time. Or a vinegar or camphor impregnated handkerchief might be held to the nose when going about. A tarred rope in the hand and a camphor bag necklace gave a hope of immunity. Others chewed garlic throughout the day, or kept the contagion away by storing it in pockets or shoes. Camps and hospitals purged their rooms with gunpowder, tobacco smoke nitre and sprinkled vinegar, or walls well scoured and whitewashed.

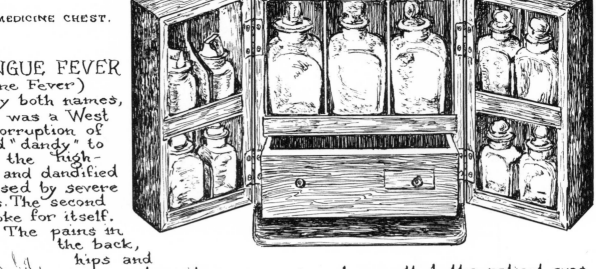

DR. RUSH'S MEDICINE CHEST.

DENGUE FEVER
(Breakbone Fever)
Known by both names, the first was a West Indian corruption of the word "dandy" to describe the high-stepping and dandified gait caused by severe leg pains. The second term spoke for itself.
The pains in the back, hips and

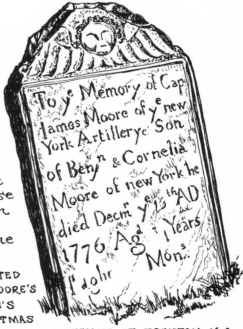

extremities were so extreme that the patient was unable to be abed. Such symptoms separated it from those of Yellow Fever, although also of viral origin and carried by the same mosquitoes.

MALARIA (Intermitting Fever)
"Malaria" or bad air was so named because of its association with the "exhalations" of marshes. It was distinguished from Yellow Fever and Dengue by periodic onsets of chills and a high fever. Different mosquitoes carried a different etiology - the Plasmodium parasites. R "The Bark"-quinine - was given for fevers in general. Here, however, was a specific for the Malaria parasites.

VENEREAL DISEASES ~ Hardly
epidemic, but any credit for their spread was given to the European soldiers. American unfortunates took the "cure" at one dollar per soldier and ten dollars for officers. The money was set aside for the purchase of clothing for the troops. R included oral salt peter and sumac roots, or a mixture of salts and turpentine. Milk was also prescribed. Hardly worth the price!

TORY~ROT ~ Last, and certainly least
of the epidemics. This was the name for those timid Americans who played no active part in the Revolution. Particularly contagious when the Britishers were hard on the heels of the patriots.

ONE OF THE COUNTLESS MONUMENTS ERECTED TO THAT DREAD DISEASE - CAMP FEVER. CAPTAIN MOORE'S TOMBSTONE IS FOUR MILES ABOVE WASHINGTON'S DELAWARE CROSSING. THE CAPTAIN DIED ON CHRISTMAS MORNING. THAT NIGHT THE ARMY SWEPT THROUGH THE HESSIANS AT TRENTON, N.J.

Since the reader is now proficient at the art of treating epidemics, consideration of a few of the routine camp problems might be in order. Except for local applications, general therapy remained the same for excessive and decreased irritability. To review, the tissue irritability of the former could be countered by bloodletting, blisters, cataplasms, formentations and clysters, medicinals and a low diet. To spruce up the debility of the latter, anodynes, cathartics, clysters, rubefacients, stimulants and a nourishing diet were required.

ROUTINE CAMP AILMENTS

INFECTIOUS ARTHRITIS (Rheumatism)

Joint pains without a previous history of symptoms, such as gout, were lumped under this classification. Exposure to cold after overheating — especially if the soldier removed his uniform and rested on a damp cold spot — predisposed the unwary to the illness. Symptoms were accelerated if one were fatigued, or soaked with rain and then wore the damp clothing without changing.

Such exciting causes were followed by shivering, thirst, uneasiness and fever. In a day or so, sharp pains bit into the joints of the extremities. If these red and swollen joints skittered here and there without localization, the disease might be driven inward. The lungs and brain became involved (this septic spread is a rarity with today's antibiotics), resulting in delusions and chest pressure.

℞ Aside from the general treatment for any excessive stimulation disease, local efforts might include the rubbing of the joints with a piece of dry flannel. If the pain persisted in any one joint, it could be countered by blistering. A happy prognosis accompanied a brick-colored sediment in the urine and profuse sweating.

18TH CENTURY CRUTCH

LEG SORES ~

Here was an unusual disease, for such ulcerations were thought to be caused by **either** increased or decreased stimulation of vessels and muscles. In the first case, injury to the skin — including such as a pinprick or mosquito bite — precipitated excessive arterial spasm and resulting skin breakdown.

℞ Of course one must go through the excessive stimulation routine. But locally, soft poultices were recommended, especially the old favorite of bread and milk. When the peripheral inflammation subsided, adhesive plasters were used to draw the edges of the sore together. Rest with the leg in a horizontal position was also beneficial.

As for the ulcers resulting from decreased stimulation, debility could be brought about by lifting heavy weights or excessive marching or standing. The blood vessels and muscle fibers were fatigued by being overstretched. The decreased tone was elevated by the usual measures. And here, gentle exercise was considered important - as opposed to the rest needed in excessive stimulation. Wounded British soldiers, after the battle of Guilford, North Carolina, recovered from any ulcerations faster when turned out of the military hospitals quickly to follow the army. If delayed on the road for but a few days, the lesions

> Bread & Milk Poultice ~
>
> Powder the bread and stir into boiling milk. Pour out and spread on a rag. Dip a knife into sweet oil or lard and smear the whole to make a solid poultice.

17

worsened and ceased healing.

    Local ℞ included arsenic, blue vitriol and tartar emetic. These were followed by astringents such as Peruvian or white oak bark, and lime water from the tub used by smithys to extinguish their irons.

IMPETIGO ~

Known as "the Itch" among the Revolutionary ranks, it " is a very troublesome distemper to armies, and immediately spreads by contact, unless the affected soldiers are separated from those who are well." The hands were usually first involved, especially between the fingers. The itchy vesicles might rupture from scratching, spreading the "itch disorder" to neighboring parts. A "disgustful crust" developed into pustules and ulcers. The closely packed campsites were fair game to this highly contagious bacterial infection.

    ℞ The body must be kept clean and the linen changed frequently. Shirts, breeches and stockings were scented with brimstone (burned sulfur) before being worn. Those tortured with the affliction bathed in water impregnated with sulfur. Ointments with a hog's lard base was supplied locally.

SMALLER WATER CONTAINERS~ DRINKING.

RIFLEMAN'S NOGGIN CARVED FROM A HARDWOOD BURL.

THE WOODEN TOGGLE WAS HELD BY PRESSURE UNDER THE BELT.

MOLDED HORN DRINKING CUP.

COWHORN CUP WITH WOODEN BASE PLUG.

HEAT STROKE

(Cold Water Disease) The Continental soldier was thought to risk death if he were to chill his innards with cold water. He who swallowed it when the body was overheated or the water chilled and of a large quantity developed fearful symptoms. In a few minutes he would develop dimness of sight, a rattling of the throat, difficulty breathing, nostrils and cheeks expanding and contracting with every respiration, the face livid in color, and cold extremities. Collapse and an imperceptible pulse followed, and the disease ended in death in four or five minutes "unless relief is speedily obtained." Clearly, here was a debility resulting from the long action of heat on the body. The skin and stomach were precipitated by the exciting cause~ cold water.

WOODEN MUG CARVED FROM HARDWOOD BLOCK.

18

℞ ~ Only one ~ if "speedily obtained," was a teaspoon to a tablespoon of liquid laudanum. Prophylaxis ~ Grasp the vessel for a few minutes or longer with both hands. Not only would the body heat be extracted, but the water would also be warmed.

DROWNING

~ Breathing water was as dangerous as drinking it cold. Here are several Eighteenth Century solutions for such an emergency.

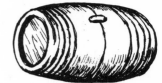

ARMY CANTEENS

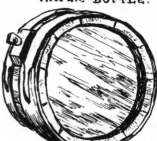

LATHE-TURNED HOLLOW WATER BOTTLE.

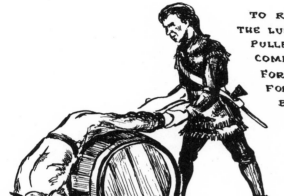

TO REMOVE WATER FROM THE LUNGS, THE BODY WAS PULLED BACK. ITS WEIGHT COMPRESSED THE CHEST TO FORCE EXPIRATION. THEN A FORWARD PUSH OVER THE BARREL RELEASED THE PRESSURE TO INDUCE INSPIRATION.

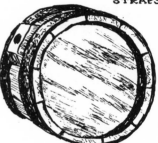

INTERLOCKING WOODEN STRAPS.

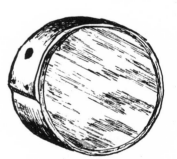

IRON STRAPS.

INVERSION OF THE BODY WAS APPARENTLY SUCCESSFUL IN MANY NEAR DROWNINGS. OFTEN PRESSURE WAS ALSO APPLIED TO THE CHEST TO EXPEL THE WATER. INSPIRATION OCCURRED WHEN THE PRESSURE WAS REMOVED.

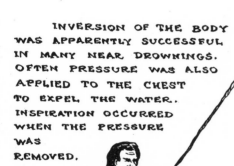

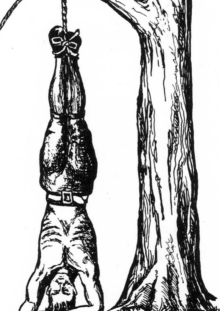

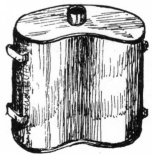

BENT AND PEGGED WOODEN SIDE STRIP.

TIN.

THE ARMY APOTHECARY

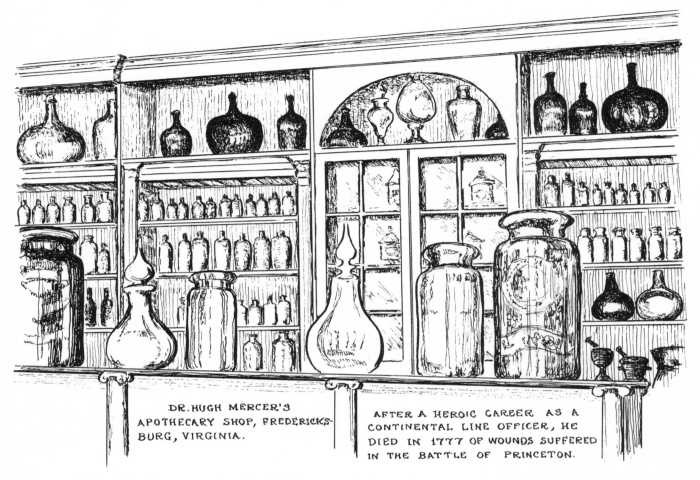

DR. HUGH MERCER'S APOTHECARY SHOP, FREDERICKS-BURG, VIRGINIA.

AFTER A HEROIC CAREER AS A CONTINENTAL LINE OFFICER, HE DIED IN 1777 OF WOUNDS SUFFERED IN THE BATTLE OF PRINCETON.

MEDICINES IN SHORT SUPPLY~ September 27th, 1776~ Col. Samuel Wigglesworth wrote this note of despair to the Committee of Safety in New Hampshire~ "Nearly half this regiment is entirely incapable of any service, some dying almost every day. Colonel Wyman's Regiment is in the same unhappy situation. There are no medicines of any value in the Continental chest and such as they are, in their native state, unprepared; no emetics nor cathartics, no mercurials, or antimonial remedies, no opiates or elixir, tincture or any capital remedy." Practicing medicine without medicine had become the usual.

Since the bulk of army "physicks" were apprentice~trained, it is of some wonder that medicines "in their natural state" were not processed by the regimental surgeons~ or collected from the countryside. Generations of Americans had done so. Every house-hold knew that potency depended on digging medicinal roots before the growing season began, collecting buds in the spring, bark during the active growing season, and seeds at harvest time. It was insured by not crushing the specimens and by fast drying away from sun and moisture.

European and West Indies medicinals were never in great supply, and now the war made the deficiency critical. The American Indian had survived nicely on local herbs~ bloodroot, wild ginger, sweet flag, sassafras, sarsaparilla, ferns, prickly pear, wintergreen, pokeweed and a host of others. The physician appreciated their curative powers, and most had apprenticed by extracting tinctures from the ever-boiling hearth kettle, powdering drugs under the pestle, and rolling pills on the slab. And, of course, they were no strangers to the imported medicinals and their preparation.

DRUGGISTS ~ Colonial druggists
(Teutonic root word "drogue" = a dry herb) were a rare breed indeed. Only the largest of cities could support their specialty of preparing drugs for physicians.

APOTHECARIES ~ The apothecaries
of yesterday were the retail druggists of today. More numerous than their druggist brothers, their shops in the more affluent towns were known by their splendid over-hanging signs. The "Pestle and Mortar," the "Ointment Pot" ~ or perhaps the "Hippocrates" ~ the "Boehaave" ~ or even the "Dove" or the "Dragon" were some of the favorites. Inside, there was no mistaking the profusion of medicinal smells from sundry aromatics, opiates, confections, conserves, purges, pills, syrups, electuaries, plasters, cerates, troches, salves and oils. Behind the counter, or in an adjacent medical-surgical office, was the owner-physician. If the shop were large enough, a chemist might be employed to prepare and dispense drugs.

Philadelphia physician Abraham Chovet, noted for his anatomical models, wrote the first prescription just prior to the Revolutionary War. By the end of the Eighteenth Century, it had become the usual method of prescribing treatment. Meanwhile, physicians hard by the apothecary shop could purchase whatever prepared medicines their practice demanded. And to those citizens inclined toward over-the-counter treatment, there were enough nostrums to boggle the mind. Made up of secret ingredients, they were sold to the gullible as a "Sovereign remedy" or "sure specific." To emphasize the remarkable curative powers, the labels often carried testimonials, and often the apothecary's signature to prove it to be the genuine article.

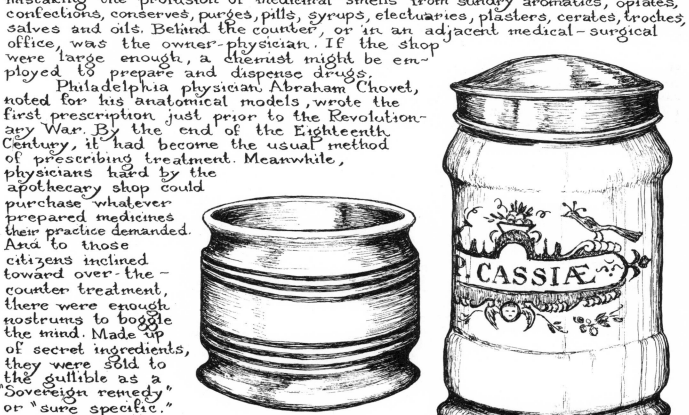

CARBOY~ THE TRADEMARK OF DRUGGISTS SINCE THE LATE 17th CENTURY. THESE PEAR-SHAPED, BLUE OR GREEN GLASS VESSELS WERE SOMETIMES COVERED WITH BASKET WORK FOR SAFER TRANSPORT. OUT-SIZED, THEY HELD 1-4 GALLONS OF LIQUIDS - FROM ACIDS TO WINE.

ENGLISH DELFT OINTMENT JAR ~ 17th CENTURY.

18th CENTURY DRUG JAR~ PILULAR EXTRACT OF CASSIA.

IT WAS CUSTOMARY FOR THE APOTHECARY TO USE SEPARATE BOTTLES FOR EACH DOSE OF INTERNAL MEDICINES. THUS THE CHARGE COULD BE INCREASED TO ONE OR TWO SHILLINGS A DOSE.

There were early rumblings that the combination of physician and apothecary was not in the best interests of curing patients. Dr. John Morgan, destined to become the second Director-General of the Continental Army Hospital, drove home the point at the commencement of College of Philadelphia in 1765. "We must regret that the very different employment of physician, surgeon and apothecary should be promiscuously followed by any one man. They certainly require very different talents." At the time, few of his fellow physicians agreed.

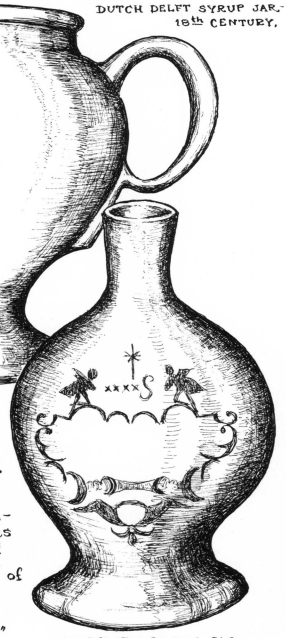

DUTCH DELFT SYRUP JAR. 18th CENTURY.

The War of Independence gave urgency to Morgan's good advice. In 1775, Congress officially recognized the value of the apothecary by creating a position on the Hospital staff. At last a specialty, the apothecary received pay and recognition equal to the surgeons. One year later, the respected Philadelphia apothecary Christopher Marshall was commissioned to prepare drugs for the troops in that area. Shortly thereafter, an Apothecary-General, equal in authority to a Surgeon-General, was authorized by Congress. The preparation of medicines had become a specialty in its own right.

ANOTHER FIRST~ Dr. William Brown, Physician-General of the Middle Department in 1778, published in that year America's first pharmacopoeia. A tiny edition it was - thirty-two pages of Latin, crammed into a page size of two and one-half inches by four and one-half inches. Its frontispiece description was more sizable!
· · · "for the use of the Military Hospital belonging to the Army of the United States of America Adapted to our present need and poverty, which we owe to the ferocious cruelty of the enemy, and to a cruel war brought unexpectedly upon our Fatherland." A second edition appeared in 1781.

DUTCH DELFT MEDICINE JAR.

CRUDE MEDICINALS — The vegetable, animal or mineral origin determined each classification. Here are but a few of the raw beginnings that became Eighteenth Century medicinals.

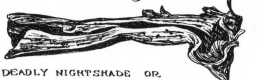

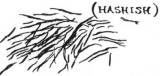
(HASHISH)

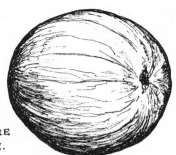

DEADLY NIGHTSHADE OR BELLADONNA. ATROPINE WAS EXTRACTED FROM THE LEAVES AND ROOTS. AMERICAN. ANTISPASMODIC, ANTISUDORIFIC.

CANNABIS INDICA OR INDIAN HEMP. THE FIBERS AND OILY SEEDS WERE MEDICINALS SINCE THE 5TH CENTURY B.C.

COLOCYNTH OR "BITTER APPLE" WAS A POPULAR PURGATIVE.

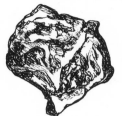

DRAGON'S BLOOD — THE EAST INDIAN FRUIT FROM A PALMLIKE TREE YIELDED A RED RESIN. ADHESIVES FOR PLASTERS.

ERGOT — A DRIED FUNGUS OBTAINED FROM RYE GRAIN. ARTERIAL AND MUSCULAR CONTRACTION.

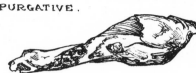

XANTHOXYLLUM ~ PRICKLY ASH BARK WIDELY USED FOR TOOTHACHE, COLIC AND RHEUMATISM!

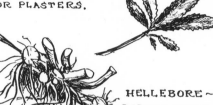

HELLEBORE ~ THE INDIAN POKE FROM AMERICAN SWAMPS AND MEADOWS GAVE A DRIED ROOT AND RHIZOME. CIRCULATORY STIMULANT, DIURETIC, CATHARTIC.

JALAP ROOT CAME FROM A MEXICAN PLANT. PURGATIVE.

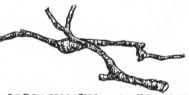

IPECACUANHA — AMERICAN SMALL SHRUB ROOT FROM MOIST AND SHADY FORESTS. EMETIC AND ANTIDYSENTERIC.

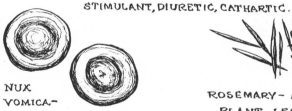

NUX VOMICA ~ "QUAKER BUTTON" THE DRIED SEED OF THE STYCHNOS NUX VOMICA CONTAINED STRYCHNINE AND BRUCINE. NERVE STIMULANT.

ROSEMARY — A MEDITERRANEAN PLANT. LEAVES AND DISTILLED OIL USEFUL.

SENNA ~ THE ARABS FIRST USED ITS DRIED LEAVES AND FRUITS.

TRAGACANTH — THE DRIED SECRETION OF A PERENNIAL SHRUB, USED AS AN ADHESIVE AND SUSPENDING AGENT.

WINTERGREEN — AMERICAN. THE LEAVES GAVE A VOLATILE OIL, METHYL SALICYLATE. URINARY IRRITANT.

VANILLA BEAN, MEXICAN. THE FRUIT OF THE VANILLA PLANT WAS FOR FLAVORING.

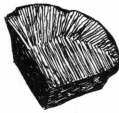

SULPHIDE OF ANTIMONY,
EMETIC.

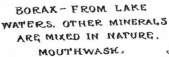

BORAX - FROM LAKE
WATERS. OTHER MINERALS
ARE MIXED IN NATURE.
MOUTHWASH.

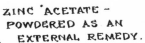

ZINC ACETATE -
POWDERED AS AN
EXTERNAL REMEDY.

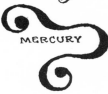

CALAMINA -
POWDERED, IT WAS USED
EXTERNALLY AS CALAMINE
LOTION.

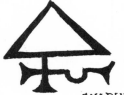

VERDIGRIS.
SHEETS OF COPPER
WERE EXPOSED TO
VINEGAR TO GIVE BLUE
HYDRATED COPPER ACETATE.
TUBERCULOSIS.

SIGNS OF THE TIMES ~ The ancient symbols of alchemy found their way into the American Revolutionary period. A few, including those for weights and measures, are familiar today.

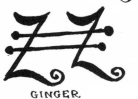

GINGER

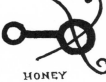

HONEY

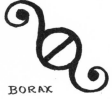

BORAX

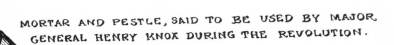

MERCURY

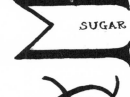

SULPHUR

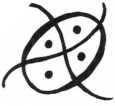

SUGAR

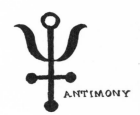

VERDIGRIS

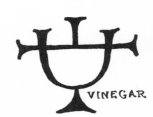

ANTIMONY

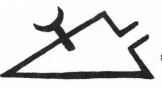

VINEGAR

WINE
SPIRIT

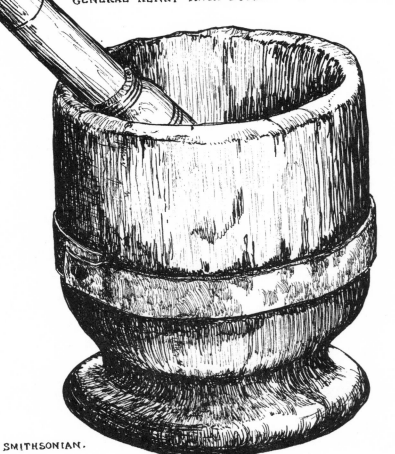

MORTAR AND PESTLE, SAID TO BE USED BY MAJOR
GENERAL HENRY KNOX DURING THE REVOLUTION.

SMITHSONIAN.

EXTRACTING THE ACTIVE INGREDIENT

1. INFUSION – Simplest and quickest. The dried medicinal was powdered in the mortar, boiled and stirred for ten minutes over the fire, then strained. The drug was then ready to drink.

2. DECOCTION – When boiling might destroy the potency, the infusion mixture was simmered.

3. TINCTURE – Those plants with oils, resins or waxes were not soluble in water. A raw dry drug of this type will actually feel oily. Alcohol dissolved these into solution after powdering in the mortar.

PREPARING COMPOUNDS –

1. BASE or active ingredient – the curative agent.

2. ADDITIVES promoted the operation of the basic ingredient. Emulsifying agents helped the union of oily and watery materials.

3. CORRECTIVES disguised the taste or moderated the activity by dilution or counter-action. Common correctives were licorice root, cane sugar, starch, and spicy pungents as ginger, sweet flag, mints, lavender, pepper, cloves and nutmeg.

4. VEHICLE – That which contained the above sub-stances and provided a usable compound.

    A. ELECTUARIES – Mixtures of powdered insoluble substances could be swallowed when mixed in a vehicle such as honey

    B. PILLS – For slower absorption and action, powdered compounds were held together with such as waxes in dry or wet form.

    C. OINTMENTS, LINIMENTS AND SALVES Varied only in the wax content of the spreading vehicle. Soap, turpentine, plant gums as camphor or myrrh, oils such as sassafras, thyme, hemlock or eucalyptole. A favorite ointment for the itch was of flour of sulphur and hog's lard. All salves contained glycerine.

BRASS MORTAR AND PESTLE OF THE EIGHTEENTH CENTURY.

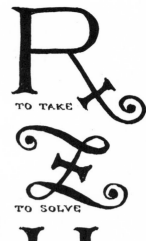

TO TAKE

TO SOLVE

TO PULVERIZE

P·I· ONE PINCH

3·I· ONE DRAM

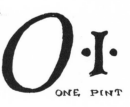

3·I· ONE OUNCE

O·I· ONE PINT

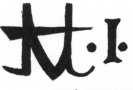

·I· ONE POUND

25

D. MIXTURE ~ A suspension of insoluble materials in a mucilaginous medium.

E. DEMULCENTS ~ An oily or mucilaginous vehicle soothing to the intestine.

F. EMOLLIENT ~ A vehicle that softened or soothed.

G. FORMENTATION ~ Hot, moist substances for application to ease pain.

F. SPIRITS ~ An alcoholic solution containing dissolved compounds.

G. ELIXIR ~ A sweetened liquid containing alcohol as a vehicle.

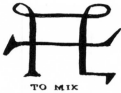

POWDER

TO MIX

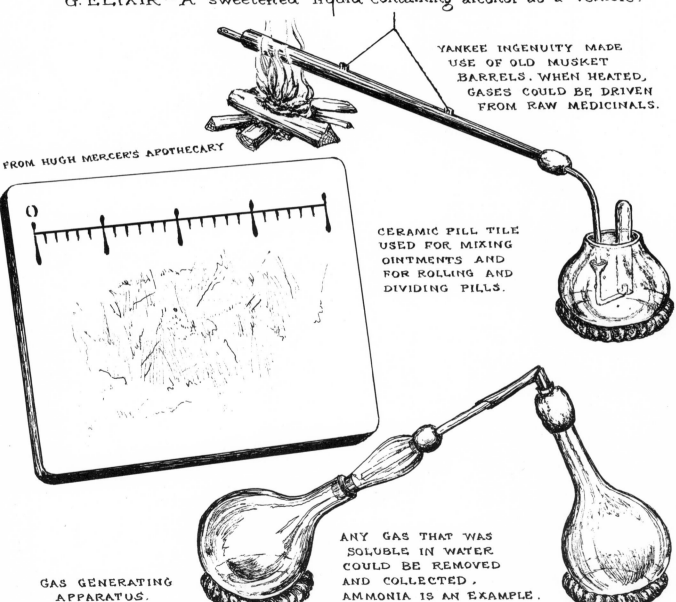

YANKEE INGENUITY MADE USE OF OLD MUSKET BARRELS. WHEN HEATED, GASES COULD BE DRIVEN FROM RAW MEDICINALS.

FROM HUGH MERCER'S APOTHECARY

CERAMIC PILL TILE USED FOR MIXING OINTMENTS AND FOR ROLLING AND DIVIDING PILLS.

GAS GENERATING APPARATUS.

ANY GAS THAT WAS SOLUBLE IN WATER COULD BE REMOVED AND COLLECTED. AMMONIA IS AN EXAMPLE.

SURGERY

In his "Travels Through North America" in 1781, the Marquis de Chastellux noted: "I make use of the English word doctors, because the distinction of surgeon and physician is as little known in the Army of Washington as in that of Agamemnon. We read in Homer that the physician Macaon himself dressed the wounds…. The Americans conform to the ancient custom and it answers very well."

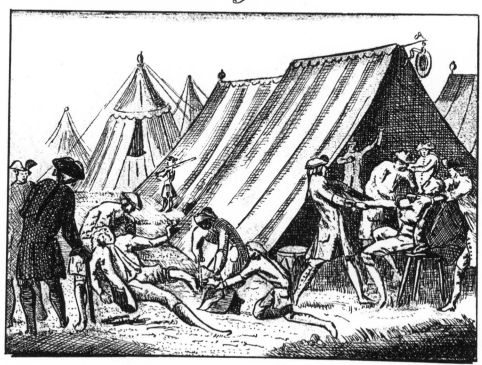

THE ARMY SURGEON AT WORK.
FROM VON FLEMING'S "DER VOLLKOMMENE TEUTSCHE SOLDAT," LEIPZIG, 1726.

When the soldier shouldered his musket, he marched into a red-coated world of trauma. Continental Army doctor-physicians took on their role as doctor-surgeons. Militia reinforcements would be called up. (I know of no battle that lacked militia assistance), along with their regimental surgeons. Because of the varied abilities of the latter, Director-General Morgan drew up the following regulations for better efficiency.

    1. Dress your wounded behind a hill 3000-5000 yards to the rear of the battlefield.

    2. Regimental surgeons are stationed with their militiamen when in a fort or a defense line.

    3. Give emergency care only. In the heat of battle, amputation or any capital operation is best avoided.
Duties include:

    – Stop the bleeding with lint and compresses, ligatures or tourniquets.

    – Remove foreign bodies from the wound.

    – Reduce fractured bones.

    – Apply dressings to wounds. If the dressings are too tight, blood is decreased, and will increase inflammation and excite a fever. If too loose, fresh bleeding may recur, or set bones

may displace.
~ Regimental surgeons and mates are ordered to assist at the General Hospital, if it becomes overcrowded with new casualties.
~ Before battle, check with the regimental officers for men to carry off the wounded and have a supply of "wheel-barrows or other convenient biers" to carry off the wounded (most "convenient biers" referred to whatever transportation was handy, and not for the patient's convenience!)

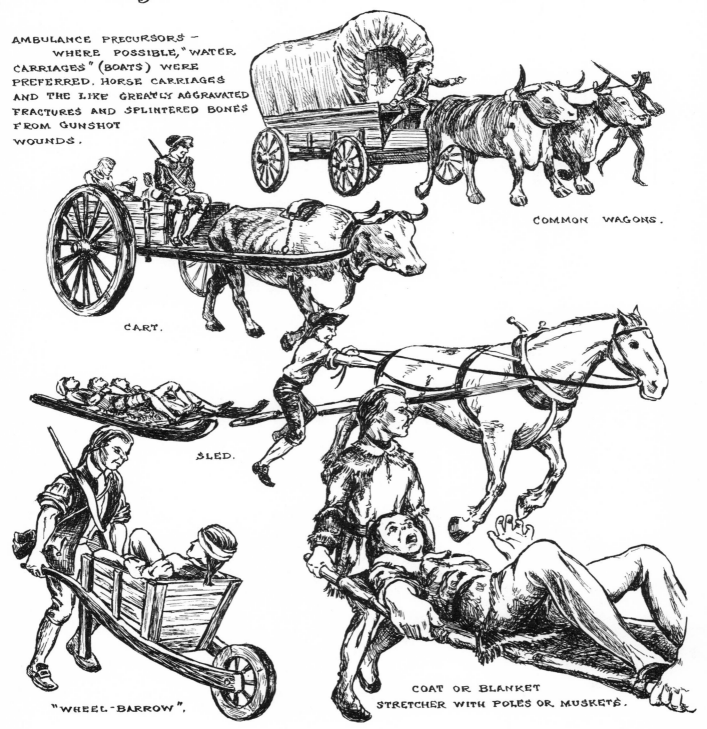

AMBULANCE PRECURSORS –
WHERE POSSIBLE, "WATER CARRIAGES" (BOATS) WERE PREFERRED. HORSE CARRIAGES AND THE LIKE GREATLY AGGRAVATED FRACTURES AND SPLINTERED BONES FROM GUNSHOT WOUNDS.

COMMON WAGONS.

CART.

SLED.

"WHEEL-BARROW".

COAT OR BLANKET STRETCHER WITH POLES OR MUSKETS.

~Each regimental surgeon should have a portable box with divisions for lint, bandages and instruments, supplied by the Director-General.

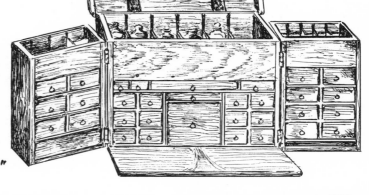

MEDICINE CHEST USED BY DR. JOSHUA FISHER IN THE REVOLUTION.

SURGICAL EQUIPMENT~

Director-General Morgan issued the following:

"A COPY OF THE ORDER AND INSTRUCTIONS, Given to the REGIMENTAL SURGEONS, In case of ACTION.

New York, July 3, 1776"

A REGIMENTAL Return of Surgeon's Instruments and Bandages, &c. now in Readiness for immediate Service, belonging to Colonel ....'s Regiment, in Brigadier General ....'s Brigade, encamped at ...., July 3, 1776.

Names of the Surgeon and Mate, and the dates of their commission.	Instruments for use	Number & kind of Bandages &c. Ligatures, &c.	Old Linnen and other implements
Surgeon. Mate.	Amputating Instruments. Trepanning, do. Incision knives. Pocket Instruments. Bullet Forceps. Crooked needles. Straight do. Pins.	Simple Rollers. Double do. Foliated bandages. Splints. Tourniquets. Ligatures. Tape. Thread.	Quantity of old linnen or weight of rags. Weight or Quantity of Lint, Tow, &c. Spunge. (Place to be signed by the Surgeon)

SCARCITY~ Much of the instrument list was wishful thinking at best. As with medicinals, there was a fearful scarcity. Director-General Morgan, obliged to supply the regimental surgeons with a medicine chest, requested in July of 1776 a report of surgical supplies in their possession. Dr. Morgan received answers from only fifteen militia regiments, and noted that so few responses indicated either a backwardness~ or that they were ashamed of being destitute. It was likely the latter. Among the fifteen that reported, there were but six amputating sets, seventy-five crooked and six straight needles, four scalpels or incision knives for dilating wounds or any other purpose, three pair of forceps for the extracting of bullets, half a paper with seventy pins, a dearth of bandages, ligatures, or tourniquets, and a little old linen, lint or tow, and two ounces of sponge that they had obtained from the Hospital. Since one regiment (also called a "battalion" and was the basic tactical unit in the army) was made up of five hundred to one thousand men, fifteen regiments would gobble up these few supplies at the first skirmish.

The Hospital fared little better. A letter, sent to Dr. John Warren, in charge of the Army Hospital on Long Island, was dated August 23, 1776. This was just four days before the British invasion of that island began. "Sir~ I have sent to the surgeons, desiring the youngest off duty to go to your assistance and take four mates with him, to carry over five hundred additional bandages and twelve fracture boxes. I fear they have no scalpels, as whatever I have committed to the hospitals has always been lost. I send you two, in which case if you want more, use a razor for incision knife. Let me know from time to time at Long Island.
                                                            J. Morgan."

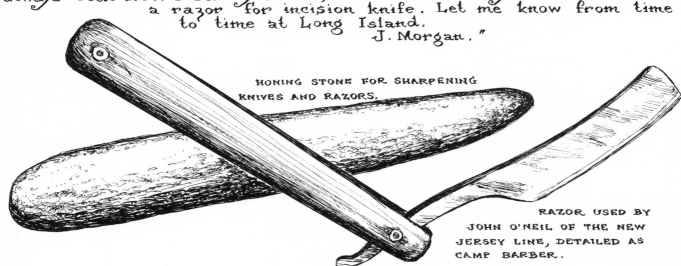

HONING STONE FOR SHARPENING KNIVES AND RAZORS.

RAZOR USED BY JOHN O'NEIL OF THE NEW JERSEY LINE, DETAILED AS CAMP BARBER.

Dr. John Jones was a Continental Army physician with extraordinary surgical skills. His book on "Plain, Concise And Practical Remarks On The Treatment of Wounds and Fractures" was published in 1775, with a reprint in 1776 and again in 1795. It quickly became the bible for both American military and civilian surgery. Many of the following surgical principles are from this excellent source.

PRINCIPLES OF HEALING

A wounded soldier usually meant a bleeding patient. Vein and small vessel lacerations yielded handily to dry soft lint compresses. The cauterizing action of styptic medicines had lost favor because of resulting tissue damage. But when blood "flows impetuously" and was of "florid color," an artery was wounded. A ligature on the vessel with a crooked needle and wax thread was the surest solution. Compression bandages or bolsters were best used if the artery were inaccessible or ran along a bone. Care was taken not to totally occlude the artery~ only enough to allow clotting. As for the aorta, any wound was invariably followed by uncontrolled hemorrhage~ and death.

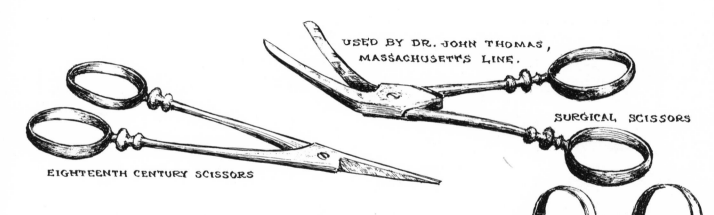

USED BY DR. JOHN THOMAS,
MASSACHUSETTS LINE.

SURGICAL SCISSORS

EIGHTEENTH CENTURY SCISSORS

STAGE OF INFLAMMATION ~

Following every break in the skin, be it a laceration, puncture or compound fracture, the surgeon could expect the dreaded stage of inflammation. On the third or fourth day following injury, the lips of the wound became hot, swollen and painful. It was believed that the symptoms of inflammation could be prevented or greatly lessened if pain could be prevented. This was done by sudorific anodynes ~ specifically, the pain-killing opium. Bleeding, gentle laxatives, warm baths and emollient poultices ~ a soothing mush of absorbent powders and watery or oily fluids ~ were adjunctive therapy; but without opium, it was felt that inflammation was inevitable.

If the course of battle delayed these measures, a different treatment was necessary. Opium could only lessen the pain, but not the symptoms triggered by the exciting cause of pain. Therefore more copious evacuations were in order, along with cooling medications a most exact diluting diet, and perfect quiet of body. And the greater the swelling and pain, the more the patient must be bled. Hopefully, the injured tissues would thereby be absorbed or converted to pus.

STAGE OF DIGESTION ~ By the fourth day,
a white matter was produced in the wound. This "laudable pus" was considered by surgeons as the best of signs. Injured tissue and vessels separated from the healthy tissue, and the symptoms of inflammation subsided. (Even after the concept of bacterial infection was known, the laudable pus concept died with difficulty, for it was still considered an excellent sign early in our Twentieth Century!)

Dr. Jones frowned upon".....the many infallable, healing balms and wonderful nostrums used by Quacks and Empericks." The two stages of healing could be jeopardized by such unprofessional remedies.

FORCEPS USED FOR REMOVING BULLETS
DURING THE REVOLUTIONARY WAR
BY DR. JOHN THOMAS.

CAPITAL INSTRUMENTS

Some surgical necessities for the medicine chest.

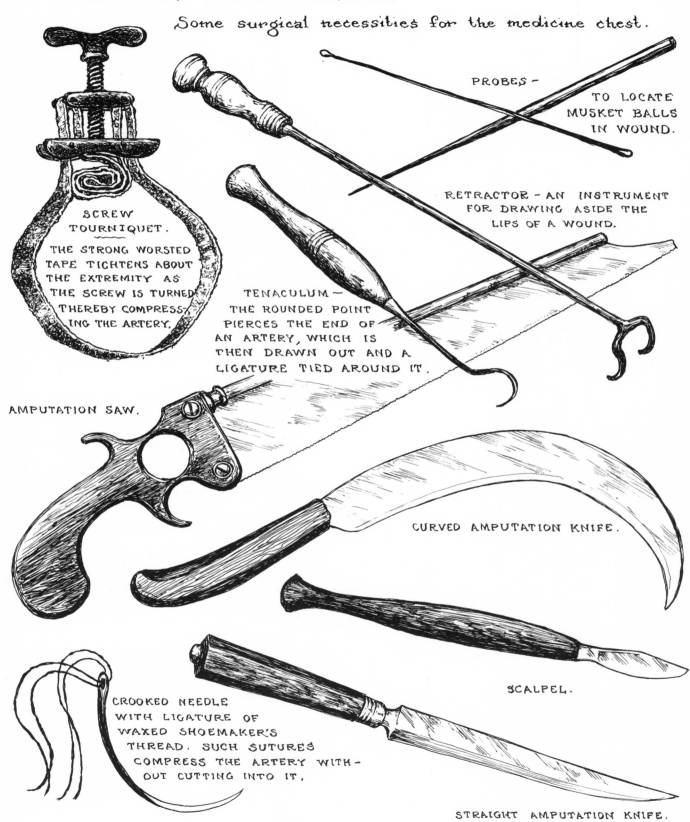

PROBES — TO LOCATE MUSKET BALLS IN WOUND.

SCREW TOURNIQUET.

THE STRONG WORSTED TAPE TICHTENS ABOUT THE EXTREMITY AS THE SCREW IS TURNED THEREBY COMPRESSING THE ARTERY.

RETRACTOR — AN INSTRUMENT FOR DRAWING ASIDE THE LIPS OF A WOUND.

TENACULUM — THE ROUNDED POINT PIERCES THE END OF AN ARTERY, WHICH IS THEN DRAWN OUT AND A LIGATURE TIED AROUND IT.

AMPUTATION SAW.

CURVED AMPUTATION KNIFE.

SCALPEL.

CROOKED NEEDLE WITH LIGATURE OF WAXED SHOEMAKER'S THREAD. SUCH SUTURES COMPRESS THE ARTERY WITHOUT CUTTING INTO IT.

STRAIGHT AMPUTATION KNIFE.

NOTES ON WOUNDS

In general, if there be loss of skin, defend the part from air with dry soft lint. A soft, mild ointment may be used to arm a pledget of tow to cover the whole. Let nature supply the loss. If a laceration heels with unequal lips, it may be later excised with a scalpel.

SIMPLE

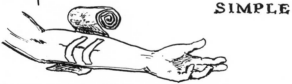

SIMPLE WOUNDS - CLOSED WITH STICKING PLASTER AND BANDAGE.

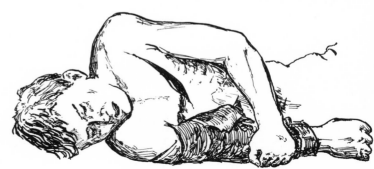

OBLIQUE WOUNDS OF BODY OR FACE MUST BE SUTURED. CLEAN OFF COAGULATED BLOOD AND FORIEGN BODIES.

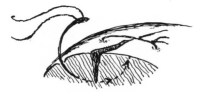

DIP YOUR NEEDLE IN OIL, AND WHILE YOUR ASSISTANT HOLDS THE WOUND CLOSED, PASS THE NEEDLE THE SAME DISTANCE EITHER SIDE OF THE WOUND AS THE DEPTH OF IT.

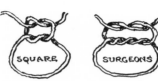

TIE EACH LIGATURE WITH A DOUBLE KNOT.

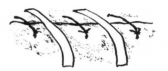

USE PIECES OF ADHESIVE PLASTER TO HOLD WOUND FIRMLY. REMOVE LIGATURES WHEN UNION COMPLETED - USUALLY 2ND OR 3RD DAY AND OFTEN AFTER TWENTY-FOUR HOURS. (PERHAPS SUCH EARLY REMOVAL AVOIDED THE STAGE OF INFLAMMATION.)

PUNCTURES

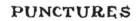

IF A CUTTING WEAPON DOES NOT ENTER A BODY CAVITY, NO TREATMENT IS NECESSARY. IF ENTERED, DILATE THE OPENING WITH FORCEPS, BLEEDING OFF THE WOUND FREQUENTLY AND AS MUCH AS HIS STRENGTH WILL BEAR.

IF PUNCTURE WOUND IS DEEP AND WINDING ~

DILATE THE OPENING TO DISCHARGE ANY FLUIDS AND TO PREVENT THE FORMATION OF AN ABSCESS.

GUNSHOT WOUNDS ~

THESE ARE MUCH MORE DIFFICULT TO CURE THAN AN INCISED WOUND. CLOTHING AND SPLINTERS ARE CARRIED INTO THE WOUND WITH THE BALL. TISSUE FIBERS AND VESSELS ARE DESTROYED. INFLAMMATION, POSSIBLY TURNING TO GANGRENE, MAY MAKE AMPUTATION NECESSARY.

SEARCH FOR THE BALL WITH A PROBE, FINGER OR FORCEPS AS LITTLE AS POSSIBLE, FOR IT WILL INCREASE THE PAIN AND INFLAMMATION. IT IS BEST NOT TO GO AFTER ANYTHING BEYOND THE REACH OF THE FINGER. (MANY FEEL THE FINGER IS THE BEST AND TRUEST PROBE.)

IF THE BALL CAN BE FELT UNDER THE SKIN, CUT AND TAKE IT OUT.

DILATE THE OPENING MADE BY THE BALL TO FREE MATTER FROM WITHIN. IF THE BALL GOES STRAIGHT THROUGH, WIDEN BOTH WOUNDS. DO NOT REMOVE ANY BALLS IF SEEN LATE. WAIT UNTIL THE INFLAMMATION IS OVER AND GOOD DIGESTION APPEARS. DRESS WITH LINT DIPPED IN OIL TO ALLOW FLUIDS TO ESCAPE MORE EASILY. WITH THE SECOND DRESSING, USE A MILD DIGESTIVE-AND WHERE THE WOUND IS LARGE, A BREAD AND MILK POULTICE.

CANNON BALL WOUNDS ~

WITH THE GREAT TISSUE INJURY, THERE IS CONSIDERABLE PAIN AND DISCHARGE OF MATTER. GIVE ONE DRAM OF BARK EVERY THREE HOURS (OR MORE OFTEN IF THE STOMACH DOES NOT REBEL). THE BARK RELIEVES THE PAIN BY TIGHTENING THE VESSELS, THICKENS THE MATTER, AND LESSENS THE QUANTITY.

TENDON WOUNDS ~

A TENDON IS THE FIBROUS CORD THAT CONNECTS A MUSCLE WITH ITS BONY ATTACHMENT. SHOULD THIS BE SEVERED, IT MAY BE REJOINED BY RELAXING THE MUSCLE AND BRINGING THE BONES NEARER.

EXAMPLE-ACHILLES TENDON TO HEEL.

FLEX KNEE TO RELAX MUSCLE.

TENDON JOINED.

EXTEND FOOT.

KEEP FLEXION WITH BANDAGE OR A LEATHER KNEE BRACE.

FOOT-LONG STRAP.

FIX A THIN PIECE OF WOOD TO AN OLD SLIPPER. WOOD PROJECTS THREE INCHES BEYOND HEEL.

NO SUTURE OF THE TENDON WILL BE NEEDED IF IT HEALS PROPERLY.

FOR ANY WOUND ~

IF THE PATIENT HAS NOT LOST TOO MUCH BLOOD, OPEN AN ARM VEIN IMMEDIATELY AND TAKE A LARGE QUANTITY. REPEAT THE BLEEDING AS CIRCUMSTANCES REQUIRE ON THE SECOND AND EVEN THE THIRD DAY.

BURNS ~

RELIEVE IMMEDIATELY BY APPLYING SPIRITS OF WINE.

NOTES ON FRACTURES

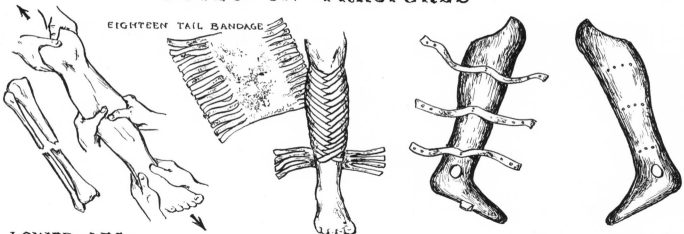

EIGHTEEN TAIL BANDAGE

LOWER LEG ~

WITH ALL FRACTURES, RELAX THE MUSCLES! PLACE THE PATIENT ON HIS SIDE WITH THIGH AND KNEE FLEXED BY YOUR ASSISTANTS WHILE YOU REDUCE THE FRACTURE.

FRACTURE AREA MUST BE SEEN, THEREFORE USE AN EIGHTEEN TAILED BANDAGE. LAP THE TAILS IN AN OBLIQUE DIRECTION. THE BANDAGE LIES SMOOTH AND EVEN, AND WILL GIVE AS MUCH TIGHTNESS AS NECESSARY.

TWO HOLLOW SPLINTS OF WOOD OR PASTEBOARD AND COVERED WITH THIN LEATHER ENCLOSE THE LEG. THREE STRAPS OF LEATHER ARE TACKED TO THE OUTER SPLINT. BRASS STUDS ON THE INNER SPLINT SECURE THE STRAPS.

WHEN SPLINTED, PLACE PATIENT ON HIS SIDE WITH THE KNEE ON A PILLOW AND HALF BENT. THE OUTER SPLINT IS PROVIDED WITH A PROJECTING REST, AND A HOLE TO PREVENT UNDUE PRESSURE ON THE ANKLE.

THIGH ~

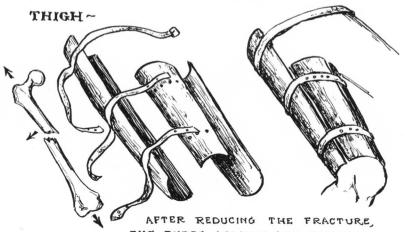

AFTER REDUCING THE FRACTURE, THE THREE SPLINTS ARE STRAPPED IN PLACE. THE OUTER SPLINT IS LONGER AND ITS UPPER STRAP IS SECURED AROUND THE BODY.

FOREARM ~

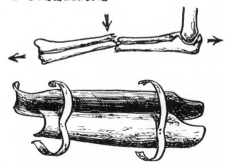

THE INNER SPLINT IS LONGER TO HOLD THE PALM. A SLING SUPPORTS THE ARM.

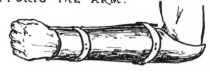

EXCEPTIONS ~ THE PRINCIPLE OF FLEXING A LIMB
TO RELAX THE MUSCLE PULL WITH BROKEN BONES DOES NOT APPLY TO:

KNEE CAP

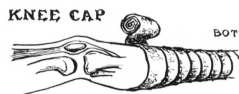

BOTH MUST BE EXTENDED BY WRAPPING WITH COMPRESS AND BANDAGE.

ELBOW

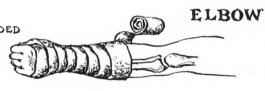

COMPOUND FRACTURES ~

YOU MUST AMPUTATE IF IN A CROWDED HOSPITAL, OR PUTREFACTION WILL SET INTO THE WOUND. BUT DO NOT AMPUTATE IF IN A SMALL TOWN OR SHIP WHERE HEALING DOES WELL. RELAX THE MUSCLES AND ENLARGE THE OPENING TO REMOVE LOOSE BONE SPLINTERS AND ALLOW BETTER DRAINAGE. REDUCE THE FRACTURE AND APPLY SOFT LINT TO ABSORB THE DRAINAGE. THE EIGHTEEN TAILED BANDAGE AND SPLINTS FOLLOW.

NOTES ON AMPUTATIONS

FOR THIS CAPITAL OPERATION, THE PATIENT IS LAID OUT AT TABLE HEIGHT, COVERED WITH DOUBLE BLANKETS AND PILLOWS FOR HIS HEAD.

LEG AMPUTATION

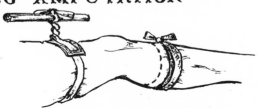

STRONG SLIP KNOT.

STICK- 4-5 INCHES LONG AND $\frac{3}{4}$ INCHES THICK.

SOLE LEATHER, 3 INCHES LONG AND $2\frac{1}{2}$ INCHES WIDE.

STRONG WORSTED BINDING 1 INCH WIDE.

FILLET & STICK TOURNIQUET.

THE SURGEON STANDS ON THE INSIDE OF THE LEG WHILE ASSISTANTS HOLD IT IN A STEADY HORIZONTAL LINE. THE SCREW TOURNIQUET OR FILLET & STICK COMPRESS THE ARTERIES. THE AMPUTATION WILL BE FOUR FINGERS BELOW THE KNEE CAP. HALF AN INCH BELOW, SECURE SEVERAL TURNS OF TAPE. CUT THROUGH THE OUTSIDE HALF, THEN THE INSIDE HALF. CUT THE MUSCLES TO THE BONE.

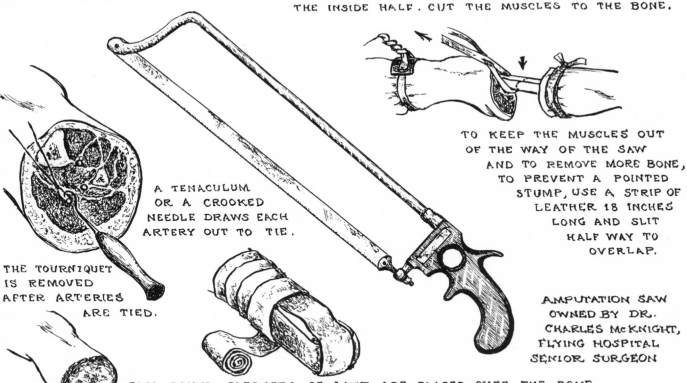

A TENACULUM OR A CROOKED NEEDLE DRAWS EACH ARTERY OUT TO TIE.

TO KEEP THE MUSCLES OUT OF THE WAY OF THE SAW AND TO REMOVE MORE BONE, TO PREVENT A POINTED STUMP, USE A STRIP OF LEATHER 18 INCHES LONG AND SLIT HALF WAY TO OVERLAP.

THE TOURNIQUET IS REMOVED AFTER ARTERIES ARE TIED.

AMPUTATION SAW OWNED BY DR. CHARLES McKNIGHT, FLYING HOSPITAL SENIOR SURGEON

TWO ROUND PLEDGETS OF LINT ARE PLACED OVER THE BONE ENDS, FOLLOWED BY A PIECE OF FINE LINEN OVER THE STUMP MUSCLES. LINT, SPRINKLED WITH FLOUR, FILLS IN THE SKIN EDGE DEFECTS. PLEDGES OF LINT AND TOW FOLLOW. LONG STRIPS OF LINEN CROSS TO HOLD DRESSINGS. A ROLLER SECURES THESE STRIPS TO THE STUMP. FINALLY, A WOOLEN CAP COVERS THE ENTIRE LEG STUMP.

NOTES ON TREPANNING

This cylindrical saw is used for an undepressed fracture of the skull to:
1. Relieve fluid pressure.
2. To allow discharge of inflammation from the brain lining (dura mater).
3. Or to prevent future mischief from a delayed hemorrhage.

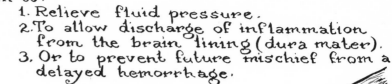

CUT DOWN TO THE BONE AND FIND THE SKULL FRACTURE. TRACE ITS FULL EXTENT TO DETERMINE THE BEST SPOT TO PERFORATE.

FIRST, PLACE THE PATIENT IN A LOW CHAIR OR LYING IN BED WITH THE HEAD FIRMLY FIXED AND SUPPORTED BY ASSISTANTS.

RETRACTOR

TREPHINE.

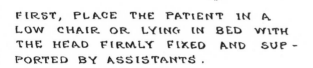

REMOVE ENOUGH SCALP AND PERICRANIUM TO APPLY THE TREPHINE. MAKE YOUR CIRCULAR CUT EQUALLY ON EITHER SIDE OF THE FRACTURE.

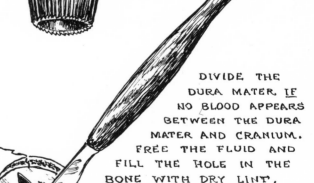

DIVIDE THE DURA MATER IF NO BLOOD APPEARS BETWEEN THE DURA MATER AND CRANIUM. FREE THE FLUID AND FILL THE HOLE IN THE BONE WITH DRY LINT.

A HANDKERCHIEF IS FOLDED IN A TRIANGULAR FORM AND PASSED AROUND THE PATIENT'S HEAD TO RETAIN THE DRESSING.

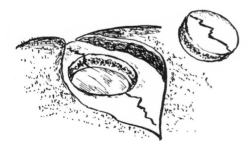

EVERY SO OFTEN, CLEAR THE TEETH OF YOUR SAW OF BONE DUST. REMOVE THE DISC AND REMOVE ANY SHARP POINTS OF BONE.

It should be noted that more die of neglect than of trepanning.

FURTHER CUTTING REMARKS

TREPHINING INSTRUMENTS.

DRAWN $\frac{4}{5}$TH SIZE.

THE FLYING HOSPITAL ~ With high hopes, Congress authorized the "Flying Camp" in June, 1776. Its proposed ten thousand soldiers were to act as a barrier to any British invasion and to supply reinforcements in the field when needed. This mobile force of militia and Continental troops was based in New Jersey, under the command of General (Dr.) Hugh Mercer. In half a year the Flying Camp was but a memory. Washington's hard-pressed soldiers rapidly absorbed the "Camp" when the British invaded New York and the Jerseys.

The Flying Hospital, designed to serve the Flying Camp and perform battlefield surgery, seemed the ideal answer for general emergency care. European armies had used Flying Hospitals for temporary battle surgery with considerable success. But in America, the Flying Hospital was a permanent and separate division from the Hospital department. Under Dr. Shippen, competition replaced cooperation. When the Flying Camp dissolved, the Flying Hospital had lost its usefulness ~ except as a stepping stone into the Director-General seat for Shippen.

"BITE A BULLET"
This was an expression of showing fortitude ~ and with good reason. Since anesthetics were unknown, patients were often given a musket ball to chew during a major operation. While being held down by the mates, it prevented him from biting his tongue or crying out.

CONTAMINATION CURE ~ Dr. James Thacher logged long and trying hours at the old French and Indian War hospital at Albany, New York. October, 1777 ~ casualties were crowding in from the Saratoga battlefield. The doctor stated that "I am obliged to devote the whole of my time, from eight o'clock in the morning to a late hour in the evening, to the care of our patients." Occasionally, the discovery of a new and successful treatment lightened the surgeon's frustrations.

"Some of our soldiers' wounds, which had been neglected while on their way here from the field of battle, being covered with putrified blood for several days, were found on the first dressing to be filled with maggots. It was not difficult, however, to destroy these vermin by the application of the tincture of myrrh."

HEADS OR TAILS? Dr. Thacher made further observations on wounds. "A brave soldier received a musket ball in his forehead between his eyebrows; observing that it did not penetrate the bone, it was imagined that the force of the ball being partly spent, it rebounded and fell out, but on close examination by the probe,

38

the ball was detected, spread entirely flat on the bone under the skin, which I extracted with the forceps. No one can doubt but he received his wound while facing the enemy, and it is fortunate for the brave fellow that his skull proved too thick for the ball to penetrate. But in another instance, a soldiers wound was not so honorable; he received a ball in the bottom of his foot, which could not have happened unless when in the act of running from the enemy. This poor fellow is held in derision by his comrades, and is made a subject of their wit for having the mark of a COWARD."

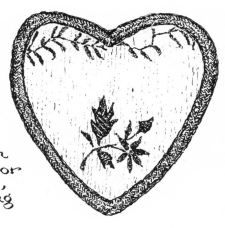

THE PURPLE HEART

~ Washington ordered the following on August 7th, 1782: "The General, ever desirous to cherish a virtuous ambition in his soldiers, as well as to foster & encourage every species of military merit, directs that when any singularly meritorious action is performed, the author of it shall be permitted to wear on his facings, over his left breast, the figure of a heart in purple cloth, or silk, edged with narrow lace or binding. Not only instances of unusual gallantry, but also of extraordinary fidelity and essential service in any way shall meet with a due reward. Before this favor can be conferred on any man the particular fact, or facts on which it is to be grounded must be set forth to the Commander-in-Chief, accompanied with certificates from the commanding officers of the regiment & Brigade to which the candidate for reward belonged, or other incontestable proof, and, upon granting it, the name and regiment of the person, with the action so certified are to be enrolled in the book of merit, which will be kept at the orderly office. Men who have merited this last distinction, to be suffered to pass all guards and Sentinels which officers are permitted to do. The road to glory in the patriot Army, and a free country, is thus opened to all. This order is also to have retrospect, to the earliest stages of war, and to be considered as a permanent one."

FRONTIER SURGERY

~ Some wilderness wounds defied the most up-to-date techniques. Scalping was one such. The Indian method was to grasp the hair with an upward pull, make the first cut below the forehead hairline, then extend to the back in a circular fashion.

Dr. Thacher related the story of a real Purple Heart candidate. "Captain Greg was immediately carried to the fort, where his wounds were dressed. He was afterward removed to our hospital, and put under my care. He was a most frightful spectacle; the whole of his scalp was removed; in two places on the fore part of his head the tomahawk had penetrated through the skull; there was a wound in his side and another through his arm by a musket ball. This unfortunate man, after suffering for a long time, finally recovered, and appeared well~satisfied in having his scalp restored to him, though uncovered with "hair."

It might be noted that such hair~raising beginnings took place at Fort St. Frédéric in 1735. There, the French first offered a substantial reward for the scalplocks of English colonists.

TEETH EXTRACTION ~ Surgery of a different

nature, but welcomed by any soldier plagued with a tooth-ache. A well~stocked medicine chest would contain a tooth extractor among the surgical instruments.

Dr. Rush noted that "When we consider how often the teeth, when decayed, are exposed to irritation from hot and cold drinks and aliments, from pressure by mastication and from the cold air, and how intimate the connection of the mouth is with the whole system, I am disposed to believe they are often the unsuspected causes of general, and particularly nervous diseases."

SCALP TROPHY ON STRETCHER.

EIGHTEENTH CENTURY TOOTH EXTRACTOR. TEETH WERE "DRAWN," NOT PULLED.

Rheumatism can be relieved by the extraction of a painful tooth.

Dyspepsia~ may improve after drawing a tooth.

Epilepsy ~ decayed teeth must be drawn and a few ounces of blood removed. If the fits recur, more blood must be drawn.

Intermittent fevers that have resisted treatment with "the Bark" may be cured by extracting decayed teeth.

Swelling, pain and ulcers of the upper and lower jaw may respond to extraction.

DENTURES were primitive and ill-fitting. Gilbert Stuart's portrait of Washington show these facial bulges clearly. Contrary to legend, he never owned a set of wooden teeth. Even with the dentures shown, appearance, eating, smiling and discomfort must have been a great trial to him.

WASHINGTON'S FIRST DENTURES WERE CARVED OF IVORY WITH HUMAN TEETH INSERTED. ONE OF HIS OWN IS THE RIGHT MOLAR.

GREENWOOD'S SECOND SET WAS OF GOLD AND WITH UPPER HIPPO TEETH AND HIPPO AND ELEPHANT IVORY FOR THE LOWERS.

DENTIST JOHN GREENWOOD OF NEW YORK MADE THESE LOWER DENTURES IN 1789. WASHINGTON'S LONE REMAINING LEFT MOLAR WAS SECURED IN THE DENTURE HOLE.

EUROPEAN MEDICINE

BRITISH AND HESSIAN~

The practice of medicine by foreign troops did not go unnoticed by our practitioners. The damning of anything British was off to a solid start when the King's troops evacuated Boston. Large quantities of hospital stores were left behind in the workhouse that served as a hospital. There, Dr. John Warren discovered that arsenic had been mixed into the medicines. It was unthinkable that the British could do such a thing, and the colonials assumed that the poisoning was the malicious work of subordinates or camp followers.

Indeed, there was a genuine admiration for the British army physician. At the Albany Hospital, after the victory of Saratoga, wounded British and Hessian prisoners received the same care as did the Americans. Dr. Thacher observed the British surgeons in action, and noted that capital operations were performed with "skill and dexterity." The German surgeons were a poor second best. They were, with a few exceptions, ".... the most uncouth and clumsy operators I ever witnessed and appear to be destitute of all sympathy towards the suffering patient."

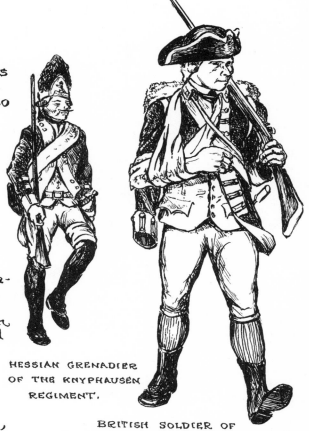

HESSIAN GRENADIER OF THE KNYPHAUSEN REGIMENT.

BRITISH SOLDIER OF LIGHT INFANTRY, 4TH (KING'S OWN) REGIMENT. AT LEXINGTON-CONCORD, BREED'S HILL, AND CHARLESTON, S.C.

FRENCH~ The chief medical officer of the French expeditionary forces under Rochambeau was Dr. Jean Coste. Foreseeing scurvy on the crossing to America, he asked for field hospitals—set up in advance—at Newport, Providence, and Papoosquash Point in Rhode Island. "Refreshments" were to include salads and cherries. Six to seven hundred soldiers and a thousand sailors developed the disease, but were cured promptly by Coste's foresight. Dysentery followed, however. The doctor felt it due to the American preference for well water over spring water. Coste made no enemies when he ordered rum mixed into the water. The doctor was also on top of a smallpox epidemic with prompt vaccination. The French troops were ready for the seven hundred and fifty mile forced march to Yorktown and the defeat of Cornwallis.

Dr. Coste soon converted the William and Mary College building at Williamsburg, Virginia, into a hospital. Dr. James Tilton, responsible for sweeping changes in the American Army hospital setup, was intrigued by the French system. He

DR. JEAN FRANCOIS COSTE.

found the patients neat and clean with every necessity – even woolen nightcaps to ward off the night chills. Almost no medicines were used, "And when they had attended my round of prescription, and saw me frequently prescribe the bark, in febrile cases, and even for the wounded, they lifted up their hands in astonishment." The French rarely used opium, and their hospital pharmacopoeia was limited to ptisans (a decoction or "tea" of pleasant taste and little medicinal value), other decoctions and watery drinks.

Dr. Tilton, with his considerable interest in better hospital care, made notes about the French ward sanitation. All manner of "filth and excrement" was thrown down a common sewer to a pit below. The structure was three stories high – from roof to ground – and it was a half hexagon of common boards. On each floor of the hospital, doors opened into this gigantic waste disposal. "This sink of nastiness perfumed the whole house very sensibly, and, without doubt, vitiated all the air within the wards." French perfume has come a long way since those early days!

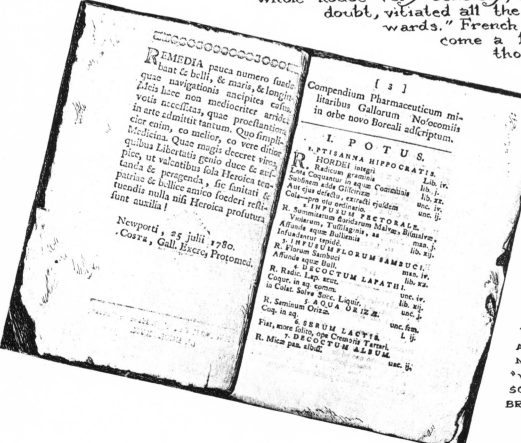

FRENCH SOLDIERS AT THE YORKTOWN SURRENDER.

DR. COSTE WROTE THIS MILITARY PHARMACOPOEIA "COMPENDIUM PHARMACEUTICUM" PUBLISHED IN NEWPORT IN 1780. ITS LATIN TEXT OF 16 PAGES GAVE GOOD ADVICE TO HIS AMERICAN MEDICAL ALLIES – "WHATEVER YOU PRESCRIBE, LET IT BE BRIEF."

HOSPITALS

SMALL HOUSE HOSPITALS ~ The independent colonist

took care of his illnesses at home. Hospitalization among strangers in a strange city had no place in his scheme of things. Almost overnight, the collision with the British around Boston created a hospitalization crisis. The regimental surgeons had no immediate problem. Minor wounds could be managed quite handily in tents or barracks. But the newly created medical department - the Hospital - had urgent need for quarters to care for the more seriously sick and wounded. Four private houses in Cambridge and three in Roxbury were hurriedly converted for hospital care. Fortunately, the British relieved the bulging hospital problems - temporarily - by evacuating Boston.

Troops and newly enlisted recruits were arriving daily in the New York City area. Director-General Morgan shortly shifted the Hospital southward to meet a new round of medical challenges. His army staff had improved with the Boston experience, and his new regulations promised efficient management of the patient. But the hospital quarters were unchanged - still the temporary quartering in local private homes as before. The Hospital's stay was no less temporary. The British invasion of Long Island and New York had begun, and the Hospital found itself in headlong retreat with Washington's troops. In the chaos of moving the wounded ahead of enemy muskets, it was clear that the Hospital must do its work deep in the countryside. Safety and permanence were vital.

BIG IS BEST? Once more distant hospital sites were

located, it seemed natural enough to build a hospital on the grand scale. America had its prototype. The British had brought the European think-big concept to upstate New York during the French and Indian Wars. At Albany, their old hospital was reopened in July of 1776. Dr. Thacher described it as: "It is two stories high, having a wing at each end, and a piazza in front above and below. It contains forty wards, capable of accommodating five hundred patients besides the rooms appropriated to the use of surgeons and other officers, stores, etc."

One month earlier, the Virginia Convention resolved to transform the splendid palace at Williamsburg, Virginia, into an army hospital. Well-appointed and staffed, the building served this purpose throughout the Revolution.

Dr. Morgan was glad enough to be rid of the small and temporary hospital homes whenever possible. On November 20, 1776, he wrote that "they ought to be floored above as to make two stories each, and have a stack of chimneys carried up the middle. Also," It is further required that bed-bunks be made, and straw be always in readiness, for the sick, and a carpenter or two be employed solely

THE PALACE AT WILLIAMSBURG.

in the business of the general hospital in making coffins, tables, and utensils of various kinds." Although the doctor was referring to the new Peekskill site, the big hospital concept applied to nearby Fishkill and other like areas.

The winter of 1776-77 saw a heavy concentration of the military around Philadelphia. The Pennsylvania Hospital was efficient and built for the job. Overflow dictated the use of the poorhouse and, for a time, a good many private houses. However, with the lessons of Long Island and New York fresh in mind, haste was made to move the sick to more distant and less populated areas. A fortunate move, for when the British marched into the city, the large general hospitals were safe enough in Bethlehem, Reading, Manheim, Lancaster and Bristol.

BIG WASN'T BEST!

Benjamin Rush observed that "Hospitals are the sinks of human life in an army. They robbed the United States of more citizens than the sword." As usual, the doctor was telling it like it was. A Revolutionary War soldier had but a two percent chance of dying in battle. But when admitted to a crowded army hospital, his likelihood of death rose to a staggering twenty-five percent! As the number of large hospitals increased, so did such diseases as typhus, dysentery, pneumonia and sundry "fevers."

① PROVIDENCE, R.I.
② NEWPORT, R.I.
③ PEEKSKILL, N.Y.
④ FISHKILL, N.Y.
⑤ ALBANY, N.Y.
⑥ HACKENSACK, N.J.
⑦ FT. LEE, N.J.
⑧ ELIZABETH, N.J.
⑨ AMBOY, N.J.
⑩ BRUNSWICK, N.J.
⑪ TRENTON, N.J.
⑫ BETHLEHEM, PENN.
⑬ BRISTOL, PENN.
⑭ PHILADELPHIA, PENN.
⑮ READING, PENN.
⑯ LANCASTER, PENN.
⑰ MANHEIM, PENN.
⑱ ALEXANDRIA, VA.
⑲ WILLIAMSBURG, VA.

PEWTER THUNDER JUG—AMERICAN.

The folly of closely packed bodies became more evident in the dark years of 1777 and 1778. The horrors of the hospital fill many a history book. When one thousand sick had to be moved from the Morristown campground in New Jersey, the large buildings of the Pennsylvania Moravians seemed a likely spot. This peaceful sect soon found their Bethlehem village flooded with the diseased. Tents were pressed into service and later the Germantown wounded added to a near impossible situation. At one point, seven hundred patients were shoehorned into the house of the Single Brethren. "Strangers Row" in the Moravian cemetery absorbed much of the overflow.

In four short months, nine of the eleven surgeons contracted typhus from the ever-present body louse. Of the two hundred soldiers who died in Bethlehem during that period, four-fifths contracted the disease while in the hospital. These were but a handful of the unfortunates that Director-General Shippen had ignored.

SMALL HOSPITALS IN FAVOR~ War accelerates changes.

With large hospital deaths skyrocketing, Dr. James Tilton stepped forward with his uncommon common sense. He noted that "...it would be shocking ... to relate the history of our General Hospital in the years 1777 and 1778 when it swallowed up at least one half of our army owing to a fatal tendency in the system to throw all the sick of the army into the general hospital, whence crowds, infection, and consequent mortality ···· I have no hesitation in declaring it is my opinion that we lost not less than ten to twenty of camp disease for one by weapons of the enemy."

During the severe winter at Morristown, Tilton designed his hospitals along the Indian wigwam design.

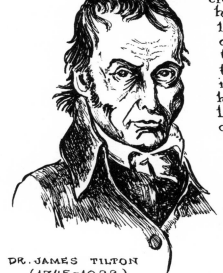

DR. JAMES TILTON
(1745-1822)

THE WARRIOR FIRST SCRATCHED OUT A ROUGH CIRCLE OF BETWEEN TEN AND SIXTEEN FEET IN DIAMETER. EACH SAPLING WAS IMPLANTED EVERY TWO OR THREE FEET ALONG THE OUTLINE, EACH WAS BENT TO MEET ITS OPPOSITE, THEN LASHED TOGETHER WITH STURDY STRIPS OF WALNUT BARK. THE TOP OF THE DOME REACHED TO BETWEEN SIX AND EIGHT FEET. AN OPENING PROVIDED FOR THE SMOKE FROM THE CENTER FIREPLACE. BEDS WERE LASHED TO THE INTERIOR WALLS AND SUPPORTED BY FORKED STICKS. A COMFORTABLE DWELLING, ONCE THE CAT-O-NINE TAIL MATS OR BARK COVERINGS WERE IN PLACE.

This Indian prototype became the new army hospital design. Dr. Tilton directed that it be built as follows: "The fire was built in the midst of the ward, without any chimney, and the smoke circulating round about passed through an opening about four inches wide in the ridge of the roof. The common surface of the earth served for the floor. The patients laid with their heads to the wall round about, and their feet were all turned to the fire. The wards were thus completely ventilated."

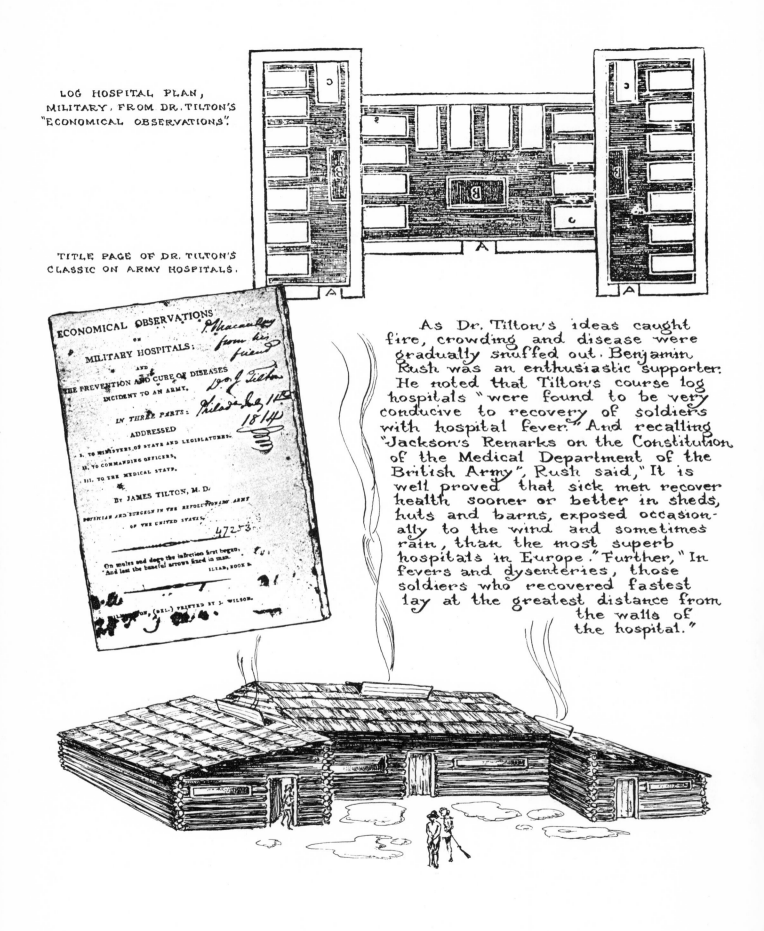

LOG HOSPITAL PLAN, MILITARY, FROM DR. TILTON'S "ECONOMICAL OBSERVATIONS".

TITLE PAGE OF DR. TILTON'S CLASSIC ON ARMY HOSPITALS.

As Dr. Tilton's ideas caught fire, crowding and disease were gradually snuffed out. Benjamin Rush was an enthusiastic supporter. He noted that Tilton's course log hospitals "were found to be very conducive to recovery of soldiers with hospital fever." And recalling "Jackson's Remarks on the Constitution of the Medical Department of the British Army", Rush said, "It is well proved that sick men recover health sooner or better in sheds, huts and barns, exposed occasionally to the wind and sometimes rain, than the most superb hospitals in Europe." Further, "In fevers and dysenteries, those soldiers who recovered fastest lay at the greatest distance from the walls of the hospital."

Dr. Tilton's booklet showed the obvious advantages of his hospital hut - then made the rather surprising statement "...that tents are in all cases to be preferred to enclosed buildings." Certainly the

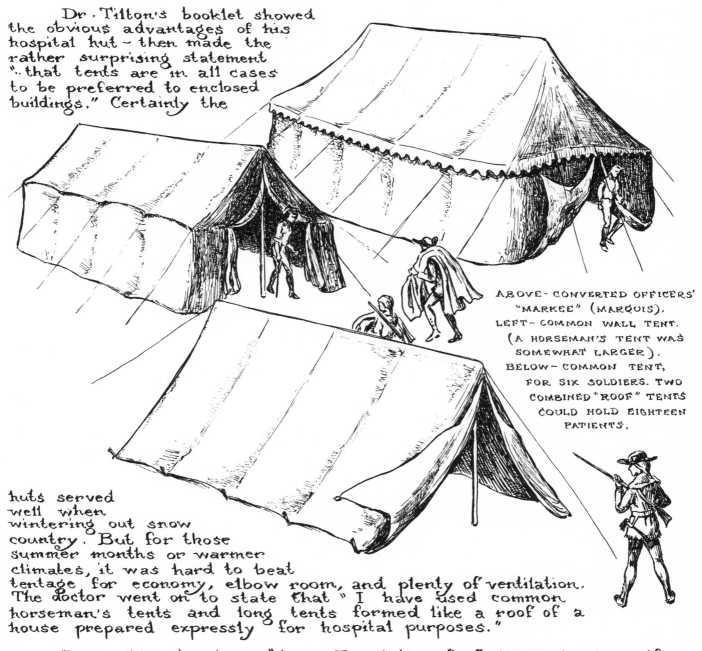

ABOVE - CONVERTED OFFICERS'
"MARKEE" (MARQUIS).
LEFT - COMMON WALL TENT.
(A HORSEMAN'S TENT WAS
SOMEWHAT LARGER).
BELOW - COMMON TENT,
FOR SIX SOLDIERS. TWO
COMBINED "ROOF" TENTS
COULD HOLD EIGHTEEN
PATIENTS.

huts served well when wintering out snow country. But for those summer months or warmer climates, it was hard to beat tentage for economy, elbow room, and plenty of ventilation. The doctor went on to state that "I have used common horseman's tents and long tents formed like a roof of a house prepared expressly for hospital purposes."

Baron Von Steuben's "Army Regulations" of 1780 gave specifics on these hospital tents. "There is nothing which gains an officer the love of his soldiers, more than his care of them, under the distress of sickness; it is then he has the power of exerting his humanity, in providing them every comfortable necessity, and making their situation as agreeable as possible.

"Two or three tents should be set apart in every regiment, for the reception of such sick, as cannot be sent to the general hospital, or whose cases may not require it; and in every company shall be constantly furnished with two sacks, to be occasionally filled with straw, and serve as beds for the sick. These sacks to be provided in the same manner as clothing for the troops, and finally, issued by the regimental clothier, to the captain of each company, who shall be answerable for the same.

"When a soldier dies, or is dismissed from the hospital, the straw he lay on is to be burnt, and the bedding well washed and aired before another is permitted to use it."

HOSPITAL DISCIPLINE ~

Crusading Benjamin Rush had other hospital improvements in mind. Independent Yankee patients were in the habit of coming and going as they pleased, often buying rum or improper foods from outside sources, occasionally "borrowing" foodstuff and clothing from nearby civilians, and disruptive of the hospital routine by quarreling among themselves or disobeying the nurses and surgeons. Rush championed the British system. In due course, an officer and guards controlled such unsoldierly conduct in each hospital. Meanwhile, a military inspector kept watch for such infractions, and reported such to the Commander-in-Chief himself. The saving of lives and Continental dollars through better discipline was inevitable.

CORPS OF INVALIDS ~

Illness had riddled the army ranks, and in 1777, Congress resolved to use these invalids for garrison duty rather than discharging them from service. All soldiers on Continental half pay were to be transferred by the regimental commander to the Corps of Invalids in Philadelphia. This highly commendable action gave the soldier, although lacking a limb or like disability, a sense of worth while continuing in the service of his country. Wounded officers, unfit for field duty, were also accepted ~ with stipulations. Not only must they present a certificate from their Continental physician, but also must have served with honor and be of good character as both soldier and citizen. The Corps not only served as a useful reservoir of experience, but also a school for improving military knowledge and discipline in the American army.

CONVALESCENT HOSPITALS ~

September, 1776 ~ Connecticut was acutely aware "...that many of the troops from this State are returning home sick and wounded, and that they are exposed to suffer for want of proper accommodations and refreshments." Upon recommendation to the Assembly by the Governor and the Council of Safety, the first convalescent hospitals in the United States came into being. Small hospitals were established in every town from New Haven to King's Bridge, New York. Local selectmen, working with state funds, sought out likely structures in their own back yard. It was a timely effort, for the dispirited and disabled from the Long Island ~ New York retreat would have need of such hospitable havens.

A chief surgeon or director was appointed by the state to supervise the hospital network, the surgeons on duty and the distribution of supplies. Four hundred bed sacks, four hundred shirts, four hundred blankets and eight hundred sheets were also supplied "...for the reception and relief of such soldiers from this State as shall serve the Continental Army, and such of the militia from this State as may from time to time join said army during the present war." These recuperation centers, uncrowded and with a hometown atmosphere, returned many a good soldier to the ranks of Washington's army.

DOLPHINS = "C"

LIGHT INFANTRY

CONNECTICUT REGIMENTAL BUTTONS.

AN OUNCE OF PREVENTION

Since the ill soldier was often a marked man, his physician stalled death as best he could. The futility of it all must have drained the spirits of those who labored in the hospital wards. If only the "contagions" could be stopped before they began, there was yet hope for Washington's dwindling ranks. Prophylaxis became the cry. As the war progressed, the army rank and file became impressed by the benefits of hygiene and sanitation. This awareness must rank as the major medical advance of the Revolutionary period.

Three publications helped to spread the word. Dr. John Jones, in his "Practical Remarks on the Treatment of Wounds and Fractures", included military hygiene in "A Short Appendix." The same year, 1776, Baron van Swieten's "The Diseases Incident to the Armies with the Method of Cure" was published. Its medical guidelines were as valued by the physician as Dr. Jones' booklet was to the surgeon.

The third voice – indeed, the crusading spirit of preventative medicine in the Revolution – was that of Dr. Benjamin Rush. He was one of the four physician signers of the Declaration of Independence and Physician-General of the Middle Department of the Continental Army. Called "Dr. Froth" by his contemporaries, he championed the British system, threw barbs at Shippen, was a keen observer of all things medical, and an outspoken enemy of society's ills. His classic broadside, entitled "To the Officers in the Army of the United American States: Directions for Preserving the Health of Soldiers," was printed in 1777. It was again published the following year, again in 1808, at least twice during the Civil War, and as late as 1908 in "The Military Surgeon." A large part of the following is from his pen.

PERSONAL HYGIENE

SKIN – Hands and face should be washed at least once daily, and the entire body two or three times weekly. Baron van Swieten was emphatic. "Neatness cannot be too much insisted on. Soldiers should wash hands, face and feet, and if the season permits, they should bath as much as possible in running water."

SHAVING – Since every soldier must appear clean-shaven for morning parade, the regimental barber did his superficial surgery the night before. Stubble was to be removed at least three times weekly. The barber supplied his own razors and soap, and

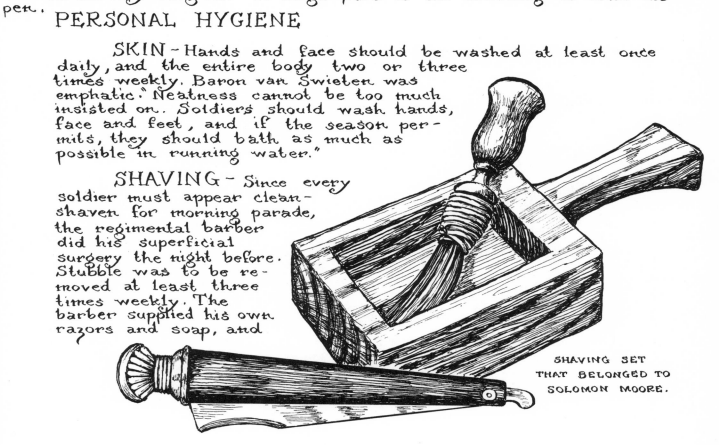

SHAVING SET
THAT BELONGED TO
SOLOMON MOORE.

the soldier supplied the payment. Apparently some saved their money, for occasionally the inspecting officers noted that the men appeared "unshaved, unpowdered, or with powder slovenly put on."

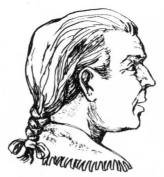

SHORT AND PLAITED.

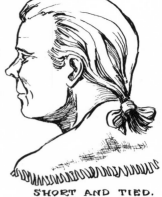

SHORT AND TIED.

HAIR ~ This was another chore for the camp barber - cutting, dressing **and** saving all the camp fat and grease that he could salvage. The amount was considerable, for half a pound of "rendered tallow" was needed for every one hundred soldiers before a general inspection.

Rush was well aware that a soldier's duty gave little time for fussing with such frills as side locks and plaited long hair. Further, it harbored perspiration and disease. He suggested that the hair be thinned and worn short at the neck - with daily combing and dressing. It would still be plaited or tied as favored by the Continentals.

Since short hair was the order of that day, the Colonel of the First South Carolina Line asked that his officers also conform to set a proper example. His orders of 1778 added that "However some of the men may prize effeminate length of hair, short hair is certainly better for actual service." Two hundred years later, the army still had its problems in dealing with long-haired servicemen.

In garrison, the soldier powdered his hair daily to look crisp and tidy.

LONG, SIDE LOCKS AND PLAITED ~ AND NOT APPROVED.

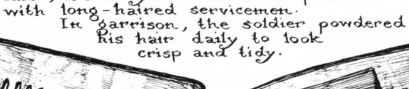

BRITISH BRASS COMB.

AMERICAN ~ BRASS.

This crop-dusting took two pounds of flour for every one hundred men. Perhaps the hungry in the ranks would have preferred it in his bread and not on his head, but a soldierly appearance was a great morale booster. Officers were required to powder when on guard duty and for ceremonies.

PROPER DRESS ~ The hunting or rifle shirt was described by Washington : "No dress can be cheaper, nor more convenient, as the wearer may be cool in warm weather and warm in cool weather by putting on undercloaths which will not change the outward dress, Winter or Summer ~ Besides it is a dress justly supposed to carry no small terror to the enemy, who think every such person is a complete marksman."

Dr. Jones recommended that a short linen coat or waistcoat with sleeves be worn under the shirt in hot weather, while flannel waistcoats did the best service on frosty days. Warm watch coats were best for sentinel duty.

Dr. Rush had his own mind on the subject. He felt that the linen hunting shirt absorbed perspiration quite handily. When mixed with rain, it "...could form miasmata which produces fever." Further, because the shirt concealed filth, and cleanliness was easily ignored, the linen should be changed frequently.

SHOES – Should be of thick and strong leather. Heavy sales helped keep the feet dry on soggy ground. All seams should be waterproofed by waxing.

It should be noted that the practical Yankee soldier wore footgear that could be worn on either foot. With no right or left, he could easily equalize the wear. Unfortunately for Washington's ranks, there would be a time when both shoes had been tramped into uselessness. A 1779 regimental order – likely one of many – hinted at the poverty of the American ragtags. "All men without shoes and barefooted will march in a separate column."

Indian shoes or "Mockasins" were considered much warmer than the common leather shoes.

INITIALLY, THE HUNTING SHIRT WAS WORN BY THE RIFLEMEN – AND THOSE WITHOUT UNIFORMS. ITS PRACTICALITY AND COMFORT SOON BECAME POPULAR THROUGHOUT THE ARMY. THE SHIRT WAS WORN ALMOST EXCLUSIVELY AROUND CAMP AND WHENEVER THE SOLDIER MARCHED OFF TO BATTLE. DEER LEATHER, HOMESPUN, OR LINEN COULD BE FASHIONED FROM THE BASIC SHIRT PATTERN. TO DISTINGUISH BETWEEN REGIMENTS, THEY WERE DYED SUCH COLORS AS YELLOW, GREEN, BLUE, PURPLE, BROWN, BLACK OR WHITE.

HEALTHY CAMPSITES ~ Guidelines for the soldier that still make sense:

TENTING ~ Pitch your camp on a dry spot, avoiding those with water just below the surface. Check by digging a hole or examining nearby wells.

In hot weather, cut boughs to shade the tents.

Keep tents open and well aired weather permitting.

If rainy, the tighter the tents the less the rain penetrates the canvas. Small trenches should be dug around the tent to keep the soldiers dry.

Avoid thick forests, for they prevent the wind from penetrating and make the air damp and close.

Camping by marshes and millponds or by rivers may dispose the soldier to bilious intermitting fever when the wind blows across the water toward the camp.

HEAT ~ In great heat, the soldiers on duty should avoid the sun ~ and above all, avoid sleeping in the sun.

AIR ~ Fire, wood smoke, burning sulphur and exploding gunpowder preserve and restore its purity.

BEDDING ~ Bed straw should be changed frequently, especially if one must camp on wet ground. Further, "The officers will be much benefited by spreading a waxed cloth under their bed." In fixed camps, when straw is hard to come by, straw mattresses or corn husks should be used. They can be easily aired, washed and dried.

Daily exposure of soldiers' blankets to the sun prevents the perspiration from becoming morbid.

Bedding should be raised a small height above the ground, especially wherever damp.

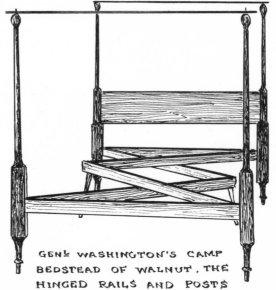

GENL WASHINGTON'S CAMP BEDSTEAD OF WALNUT. THE HINGED RAILS AND POSTS ALLOWED THE COT-SIZED BED TO FOLD INTO A TIDY BUNDLE. BED IS DRAWN PARTLY OPENED.

No soldier should sleep in wet clothes or on wet straw.

PRIVIES ~

Dr. Jones emphasized that "... no soldier should be permitted to ease himself anywhere about the camp except in the privies." At first sign of spreading flux, dig privies deeper than usual and once a day a thick layer of earth should be thrown into them.

Privies should be either in front of or the rear of the camp according to the wind direction "...which will carry off the "putrid effula."

OBSERVATIONS on health in the camps; Dr. Rush's busy notebook yielded many other thoughts on sanitation, later published in his "Medical Inquiries and Observations."

1. The army, when in tents, was always more sickly than in the open air.

2. Young men under twenty years of age were subject to the greatest number of camp diseases.

3. The southern troops were more sickly than the northern or eastern troops.

4. The native Americans were more sickly than the natives of Europe who served in the American army.

5. Men above thirty years of age were the hardiest soldiers.

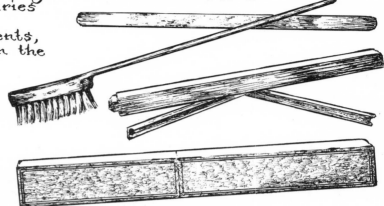

WASHINGTON'S TOILET SET. THE TOOTH-BRUSH AND TONGUE SCRAPER ARE OF SILVER, AS IS THE TOOTH POWDER CASE. IT IS DIVIDED INTO TWO COMPARTMENTS. THE CASE IS TOOLED RED LEATHER, 5 X $\frac{3}{4}$ X $\frac{1}{2}$ INCHES.

A FURTHER OBSERVATION ~ Rush's effort to prevent disease was bolstered by an unexpected and unappreciated ally - retreat. Time and again the exasperated British marched to a battle site of Washington's choosing. They received the volleys of American bullets as their rows pressed forward, only to find their quarry had melted into the countryside. While British communiques happily announced the winning of the field, the Continental Army was intact and building their resources for another hit and run. Washington was willing to lose a battle. Meanwhile, an army on the move could outdistance the epidemics that fed on the close contacts of a long encampment.

VICTUALS "...should consist CHIEFLY of vegetables."

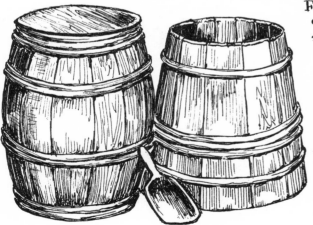

Fresh fruits and greens prevent and cure scurvy and are wholesome nourishment. Unripe and acrid fruits are very hurtful.

Avoid eating large amounts of meat. Dr. Rush noted that the southern troops sickened from want of salt provisions. Their strength and spirits were restored only with salted meat. "I once saw a private in a Virginia regiment throw away his ration of choice beef, and give a dollar for a pound of salted bacon."

MEAT BARREL AND SALT PORK BARREL. FRESH PORK WAS STORED IN A BRINE OF SALT AND WATER.

Bread must be well baked and of good pure flour. Very dangerous distempers are caused by musty or spoiled bread.

Wash cooking vessels carefully after using.

(As a general rule, the troops received a greater variety of rations when camping near large cities. In such days of plenty, as when the army camped at Cambridge in 1775, corned beef and pork were available four days a week, salted fish one day, and fresh beef for two days. The following victuals have been noted in various regimental orders — corned beef and pork, salted fish, fresh beef, rice, Indian meal, hog's lard, beans, peas, potatoes, onions, turnips, bread and hard bread. This mouth-watering array was but a memory on the march. Then, only hard bread and salt pork were on the menu.)

WATER ~ Drinking water must be pure. Do not draw river water near the banks.

To check the purity, let a few drops of oleum tartari per deliquium fall into a glass of water. If impure, it becomes thick and cloudy, while purer water gives only a small cloud.

Correct bad water by mixing six ounces of vinegar with three quarts of water. This "will render the drink even more agreeable." Water may also be rendered less hurtful by steeping it in some pieces of root calamus aromaticus." This root is found everywhere, especially in marshy places, where commonly the water is worst."

"NOTHING" is more hurtful to the soldier, when heated with work, than to strip, expose himself to cool air and then drink greedily of cold water. Well water is especially cold. River water is better, for the sun prevents it from becoming cold.

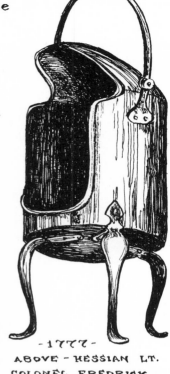

CAST IRON KETTLE FROM THE BENNINGTON, VT. BATTLE, 1777.

-1777-
ABOVE - HESSIAN LT. COLONEL FREDRICK BAUME'S CAMP STOVE, TAKEN AT HIS SURRENDER NEAR BENNINGTON, VERMONT.

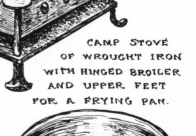

CAMP STOVE OF WROUGHT IRON WITH HINGED BROILER AND UPPER FEET FOR A FRYING PAN.

GEN'L WASHINGTON'S COOKING POT WITH COVER.

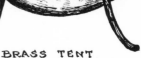

BRASS TENT COOKING POT WITH IRON LEGS.

SPIRITS OF '76

Rum "...leaves the body languid and more liable to be affected with heat and cold afterward. Happy would it be for our soldiers if the evil ended here!" By so wearing away resistance, Rush felt the soldier fell easy prey to fevers, fluxes, jaundices and the like.

General Washington also had his misgivings, but he had army discipline more in mind. With his army pouring in for the defense of New York in 1776, the evils of the big city became a problem. So big, in fact, that he gave one of the first "Off Limits" orders in American military history.

"The gin shops and other houses where liquors have been heretofore retailed within or near the lines (except the house at the Two Ferries) are strictly forbidden to sell any for the future to any soldier in the Army and the inhabitants of said houses near the lines are immediately to move out of them; they are to be appropriated to the use of the troops.

"If any soldier of the Army shall be found disguised with liquor, as has been too much the practice heretofore, the General is determined to have him punished with the utmost severity, as no soldier in such situation can be either fit for defence or attack. The General orders that no sutler in the army shall sell to any soldier more than one half pint of spirit per day."

Still, that half pint went a long way toward "raising the spirits" during those hard and hungry campaigns. The sutler - the army's civilian storekeeper sold his liquid tranquilizers of home-brewed spirits, gin, rum, cordials, common beer, strong beer, and that old back-country favorite, "cyder-royal." A bonus went to those soldiers who completed such fatiguing duties as guard duty, heavy labor, or long marches. Taking exception to his General Orders, Washington saw to it that the army stores gave a ration of alcohol after the soldier had been exposed to stress.

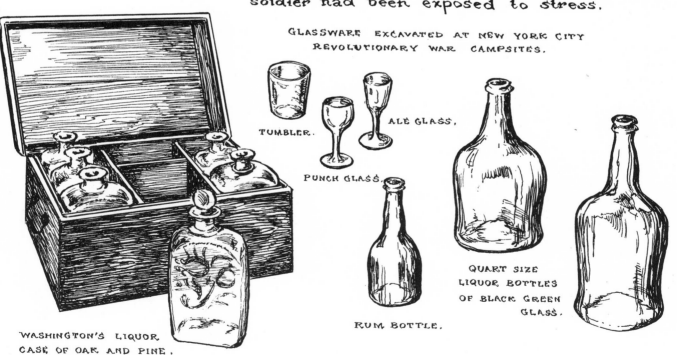

GLASSWARE EXCAVATED AT NEW YORK CITY REVOLUTIONARY WAR CAMPSITES.

TUMBLER.

PUNCH GLASS.

ALE GLASS.

RUM BOTTLE.

QUART SIZE LIQUOR BOTTLES OF BLACK GREEN GLASS.

WASHINGTON'S LIQUOR CASE OF OAK AND PINE. LENGTH 18", WIDTH 12", HEIGHT 13".

STRESSES IN BATTLE

First hand-reports of the stresses faced by the Revolutionary War soldier were documented in Benjamin Rush's "Medical Inquiries and Observations":

Thirst was a common sensation at the first onset of battle, even on such a remarkably cold day as that of January 3rd 1777. The Battle of Princeton was underway. The soldiers also felt a glow of heat, so general that it was even felt in both ears.

If fighting was hot work in chilly weather, it was doubly so on a summer's day. At the Battle of Monmouth, June 28, 1778, the temperature broiled to 90° Fahrenheit. Many soldiers were found dead without wounds, for their "emotions" had excited body heat that added to the excessive temperatures of the day.

Soldiers bore operations after the battle with much more fortitude than at any time afterward.

Pulmonary consumption was sometimes cured by the hardships of camp life.

Dr. Blane, after a study of seamen's diseases, found that scurvy and other illnesses were checked by the prospect of a naval engagement. British seamen, after the victory over the French fleet on April 12, 1782, had an "extraordinary healthiness." The effect of victory on the mind was verified by Rush. Fifteen hundred Philadelphia militia joined Washington's battered army in December of 1776 and helped take the Hessians at Trenton. Although they lived in tents or in the open during those six foul weeks of December and January, there were but two instances of sickness and only one death. Such great good health was due to the vigor infused into the body by the Trenton victory "...having produced insensibility to all the usual remote causes of diseases."

Militiamen who enjoyed good health on a campaign often became ill upon returning home. "I knew one instance of a militia captain, who was seized with convulsions the first night he lay on a feather bed, after sleeping several months on a mattress, or upon the ground." The system was toned up by a sense of danger and other invigorating aspects of a military life, wrote Dr. Rush.

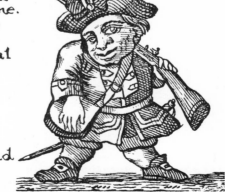

"Nostalgia" (homesickness) was a frequent disease in the army, especially the New England states. However, this ceases with danger or action. "Of this General Gates furnished me with a remarkable instance in 1776, soon after his return from the command of a large body of regular troops and militia at Ticonderoga. From the effects of the nostalgia, and the feebleness of the discipline which was exercised over the militia, desertions were very frequent and numerous in his army, in the latter part of the campaign; and yet during the THREE WEEKS in which the general expected every hour an attack to be made upon him by General Burgoyne, there was not a single desertion from his army, which consisted at that time of 10,000 men.

"The patience, firmness and magnanimity, with which the officers and soldiers of the American army endured the complicated evils of hunger, cold and nakedness, can only be ascribed to an insensibility of body produced by an uncommon tone of mind, excited by love of liberty and their country."

STRESSES ON FRIEND AND ENEMY

The winter of 1774-75 was a period of uncommon anxiety in America. Everyone awaited the results of a petition to the King which would result in reconciliation or a "civil war with all its terrible and distressing circumstances." During that time, Philadelphia saw a heavy number of apoplectic cases. The fit that deprived Congress of the considerable talents of Peyton Randolph, was due in part to the pressures of those uncertain times, so it was said.

Many sick or of "delicate habits" were restored to health by the change of place or occupation that had exposed them to the trials of war. This was especially true of hysterical women who were anxious for success in the war. Passions also had their influence on diseases ~ love, jealousy, grief or complaints. "An uncommon cheerfulness prevailed everywhere among the friends of the Revolution. Defeats, and even the loss of relations or property, were soon forgotten in the great objects of the war," wrote Rush.

The Revolution brought forth a rash of fruitful marriages. The population of the United States had more births during that period than the same number of years since the settlement of the country.

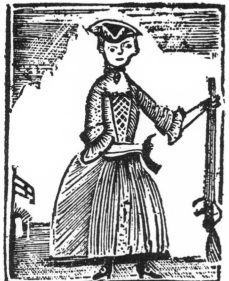

WOODCUT FROM A NEWBURYPORT MASS?? BROADSIDE. NOT ALL OUR PATRIOTIC WOMEN WERE OF "DELICATE HABITS"!

Emotion claimed its victims, such as the aged door-keeper of Congress. The ancient fellow expired on the spot when he heard of the capture of Lord Cornwallis's army. Political joy is one of the strongest emotions that can agitate the mind, observed Dr. Rush.

"Protection fever" - a term applied to those who swore allegiance to Britain in order to protect their estates. Many died when the redcoats evacuated their area, as at Charleston. This was felt due to the neglect from their former friends who supported the revolt. Rush concluded that "From the causes which produced this hypochondriasis, I have taken the liberty of distinguishing it by the name of revolutiana."

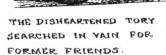

THE DISHEARTENED TORY SEARCHED IN VAIN FOR FORMER FRIENDS.

SEA SURGEONS

The Navy Department began hostilities with Britain much like the Medical Department - entirely from scratch. It very nearly ended that way. Of the sixty-four Continental vessels commissioned, but seven were still in service by 1782. American privateers swarmed out to fill the gap - close to eight hundred of them. Washington had his answer to the King's strangle hold on the high seas.

EIGHTEENTH CENTURY ANCHOR.

COOKBOOK MEDICINE ~ Finding the answer for
medical coverage was more difficult. The larger Continental ships were well staffed. But those of lesser size and the privately owned privateering vessels found physicians in scant supply. Then the art of healing became the captain's responsibility - or that of one of his officers. Reading ability, not diagnostic skill, was the prerequisite. By thumbing through the medical text, the symptoms were matched, the disease discovered, and the treatment begun. For example:

PLEURISY
Symptoms - Sharp pain and stitches felt in breast and attended with fever and cough.
Remedies - Bleeding is first and chief remedy. Let 12 oz. or even more.
Flannel dipped in the formentation of No. 12 to be applied, or Plaster of labanum spread on leather or linen.
Drink No. 13 every half hour and after it a warm cupful of No. 1.
Let nourishment be light and consist of broth, roasted apples and well fermented bread. Plain barley water to drink.

"Commonly degenerates into a consumption unless means are found to evacuate the already formed pus. A small plaster is applied to the most painful place. Corrode with a light caustic and when open, care must be taken to keep up the supporation. In such a case there is reason to hope, as the resistance is the least at this place, that the matter collected will take its course and be discharged by it."

Treatment was further simplified for the novice. To avoid the jaw-breaking Latin labels that tradition had bestowed upon each medicine, the sundry vials and bottles were marked with numbers. These numbers corresponded to those listed in the back of the book under some such title as "Recipes Referred to in the Foregoing Treatise on Diseases."

No.1 Species for the pectoral decoction 3 oz.. Boil in sufficient ½ hour to steam.

No.12 Take species for emollient decoction-3 oz. Boil an hour in water; strain five pounds. Dissolve Venice soap, 2 oz.; mix for a formentation.

No.13 Take pure nitre one drachm and a half craw claws two drachams, syrups of wild poppies 2 oz, barley water 10 oz.. Mix."

Hopefully, this medicine by the numbers - and a dose of salt air ~ would bring on recovery!

SEA SICKNESS -

When the Atlantic coastline had dropped below the horizon, the sea surgeon was on his own. His world had been condensed into a rolling compartmented wooden shell. All the hazards of the closely packed shore hospitals were there, as well as medical challenges less known to landlubber medics.

Before the sailor had his sea legs, he had the misery of sea sickness to reckon with. Dr. Usher Parsons, in his 1820 edition of "Sailor Physician," which "Intended to Afford Medical Advice To Such Persons While at Sea where A Physician Cannot Be Consulted," gave interesting advice in the subject.

"With very few exceptions, this attacks all persons on their first voyages; and the degree of it is generalized inversely proportioned to the size of the vessel, it being most violent where the vessel is small, and least so in large vessels, on which the waves make but slight impression. Some persons, however, are

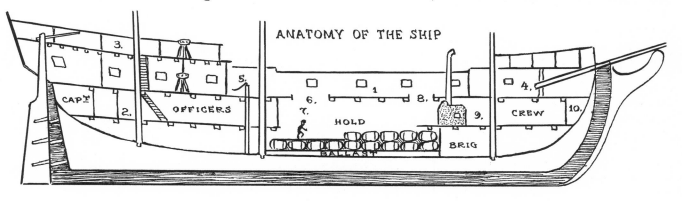

ANATOMY OF THE SHIP

1. MAIN (GUN) DECK   3. QUARTERDECK   5. PUMPS   7. CABLE TIER SHELVES   9. GALLEY
2. BERTH DECK   4. FORECASTLE   6. MAIN HATCH   8. FORE HATCH   10. HEAD

more liable to sea-sickness than others. Those in the prime of life and of a fair, light complexion have been remarked to be most susceptable of its attacks, while those of a dark complexion suffer least. The duration of sea-sickness is very uncertain, being generally not above a day or two, but in many cases it continues for weeks or even months, and there are some seamen who always suffer an attack in tempestuous weather, even after having followed the sea for many years."

Dr. Parsons goes on to note that the nausea and headaches might yield only to time — or perhaps a draught of seawater to cleanse the stomach and bowels. But in severe cases, the victim should rest his head "...on a book, or other hard substance," keep in one position, eyes closed, "...and the thoughts engaged on some interesting and agreeable subject...."

SCURVY —

Unusual weariness and pains throughout the body, numbness of the limbs, swollen legs covered with foul, black blisters, foul breath, swollen gums, teeth that loosen, turn yellow, then blacken. A ship's surgeon would quickly diagnose such symptoms as scurvy. Prevention and cure were just as familiar to the seagoing American rebels as their British "Limey" enemies. Ports in warmer climates yielded plentiful provisions of oranges and lemons. But such perishable cargo would be of little help unless the following precautions were taken:

Clear the juice from the pulp. Let it stand and pour it off from the sediment. Pour into a clean, open vessel of china or stoneware, wider at the top than at the bottom. Put this into a pan of water over a fire and let the water come almost to a boil. Continue until the juice is a thick syrup. The slower the evaporation, the better — twelve to fourteen hours should do it. When cold, cork it in a bottle for later use. When it is mixed with water to make a punch, few can tell it from fresh juice.

American farmers could also supply the navy with such tolerable scurvy preventatives as boiled and pickled cabbage, berries such as gooseberries, wild plums and alderberries, turnips and water dock. Crab-apples, apples, pears or

DRIED POTATOES — USED ON LONG VOYAGES.

A
TREATISE
OF THE
SCURVY.
IN THREE PARTS.
CONTAINING
An inquiry into the Nature, Causes, and Cure, of that Disease.

Together with
A Critical and Chronological View of what has been published on the subject.

By JAMES LIND, M.D.
Fellow of the Royal College of Physicians in Edinburgh.

EDINBURGH:
Printed by SANDS, MURRAY, and COCHRAN
For A. MILLAR, in the Strand, London.
MDCCLIII

LIND'S "TREATISE" OF 1753 — SCURVY PREVENTION FOR EVERY SEAFARER.

any other fruit could be preserved by boiling in coarse sugar. Apples and pears would keep for two or three months if they were well packed in dry, tight casks or cut up in slices and put on strings to dry.

PRESERVATION OF VICTUALS was included in the

first "Rules For The Regulation of the Navy of the United Colonies," printed 1775. Guidelines included frequent inspections of provisions. Damp bread was to be aired on the quarter-deck or poop. If any of the "pickle" or brine had leaked from a "flesh" cask, it must be replaced and the container made tight and secure. Flour and suet must not be kept aboard longer than four months.

Article 17 gave pointers on a handy supply of food for the sea-farer ~ freshly preserved in its own brine. "All ships furnished with fishing tackle, being in such places where fish is to be had, the Captain is to employ some of the company in fishing the fish to be distributed daily to such persons as are sick, or upon recovery, if the surgeons recommend

HARD TACK OR SHIP'S BREAD, 1785.

4/5 TH SIZE.

it; and the surplus by turns amongst the messes of the officers and seamen without favour or partiality, and *gratis*, without any deduction of their allowance of provisions on that account."

SICKBAY - Article 16 of the Rules stated that "A convenient

place shall be set apart for sick or hurt men, to be removed with their hammocks and bedding when the surgeon shall advise the same to be necessary: and some of the crew shall be appointed to attend and serve them and to keep the place clean." The ship's hospital or sickbay had no specific location. Generally it ended up in the forecastle (certainly in the fore of the vessel but hardly a castle). The contemporary Smollett's "Roderick Random" gave a few specifics.

"When I followed him into the sick-berth or hospital and observed the situations of the patients, I was much less surprised that the people should die on board, than that any sick person should recover. Here I saw about fifty miserable distempered wretches, suspended in rows, so huddled one upon another that not more than fourteen inches space was allowed for each with his bed

IVORY MEDICINE DROPPER.

and bedding, and deprived of the light of day as well as of fresh air, breathing nothing but a noisome athmosphere of the morbid steams exhaling from their own excrements and diseased bodies, devoured with vermin hatched in the filth that surrounded them and destitute of every convenience necessary for people in that help-less condition."

ADVICE FOR SEA SURGERY ~ NAVAL REGULATIONS.

INVENTORY ~ Be ready for any emergency. Your apparatus should consist of:

1. Capital instruments ~ keep them clean, bright, in good order and in a drawer by themselves.
2. Several tourniquets ~ Petit's screw tourniquet is most convenient, and the patient can manage it himself to stem his bleeding while awaiting surgery.
3. Crooked needles of all sizes with shoemakers' thread ligatures.
4. A large quantity of scraped (short) lint. Some mixed with flour in a bowl.
5. Double and single-headed rollers 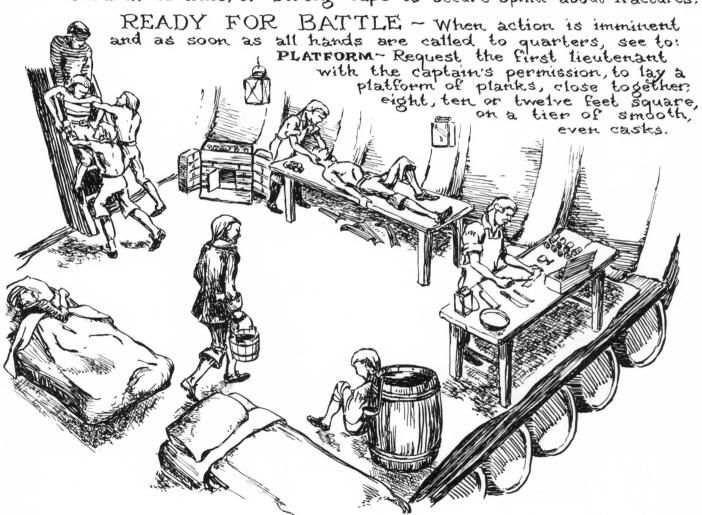 (bandages of all breadths and lengths). Bunting (woolen and cotton cloth) is used for slight wounds and contusions, while linen rollers are best used for amputations, fractures and dislocations.
6. Common needles, thread and pins aplenty.
7. Pledgets of tow (tufts of wool before spinning) of various sizes wet with water or oxycrate and dried by the galley fire or sun. By this means they will lay better together in a drawer without intertangling, and are easier to spread with any cerate (wax or resin mixed with oil, lard and medicinal ingredients), ointments or liniment.
8. Splints of all sizes ~ when ready for use, arm with tow or old linen cloth.
9. Bolsters or compresses of cloth or course tow.
10. Yards of incle, or strong tape to secure splint about fractures.

READY FOR BATTLE ~ When action is imminent
and as soon as all hands are called to quarters, see to:
PLATFORM ~ Request the first lieutenant with the captain's permission, to lay a platform of planks, close together, eight, ten or twelve feet square, on a tier of smooth, even casks.

Locate in one of the cable tiers if it is available; otherwise, set up your surgery in the afterhold. If your ship be small and has no cockpit, find a spot as near the afterhold as possible.

PREPARATION ~ Lay out your equipment as follows:

1. On one side of the platform, lay out your capital instruments, needles and ligatures, lint, flour in a bowl, styptic, bandages, splints, compresses, pledges spread with yellow basilicon or some other proper digestive, thread, tape, tow, pins, and new and old linen cloth.

2. Prepare the medicine chest with ung. basil.~c. gum. elem.~sambucin; ol. lin.~; oli~var. c.~terebinth; bals. terebinth; tinct. styp.~thaebaic; sp. c.c. per se.~vol aromat.~lavend. c.. There should be wine, punch or grog, and vinegar aplenty.

3. A bucket of water to put sponges in, another to receive blood from operations.

4. Dry swabs to keep the platform dry.

5. A water cask full of water, head knocked in, to be dipped out as needed.

6. Seamans' bedding laid side by side.

Instruct mates and assistants as to their stations.

Have the first officer quarter a number of hands in the cockpit, should assistance be needed in battle.

Send any crew, too sick to go to quarters, into the hold~or some such area out of the way~with their hammocks and bedding. The platform is only for wounded. Have a man check on the sick occasionally. In case of faintness, give them a little cordial.

Light a large number of large candles as soon as the engagement begins.

DURING ACTION ~ As the wounded come down, take care of those in the most immediate danger; otherwise, dress the wounds as they come.

Have a mate apply a tourniquet to a limb off or to any violent hemorrhage, if you are in the middle of a capital operation. The tourniquet should remain in place, ready to stop a fresh hemorrhage. Instruct the patient to tighten it, should he feel the wound bleeding before help comes.

When readying a patient for a capital operation, encourage him, promise to treat him tenderly, that you will finish as soon as possible, and that you will not cut more than is necessary. At the same time, act as though you are unaffected by their groans and complaints, but in no case, behave rashly or cruelly.

Insist that the wounded, once dressed and little hurt, return to their stations at quarters. If they lag, threaten to report them after the engagement is over. There are some dastardly fellows who have even been known to stand in the way of a recoiling gun carriage in order to go to the doctor. There is no place for cowards, including your surgical platform.

AFTER THE ENGAGEMENT ~ Give a proper diet and medicines suitable to the symptomatic fevers and such.

After seeing to your wounded, acquaint the captain of

the number of injured, the nature of wounds, and if any are likely to prove mortal. Ask him to order cradles to hold the wounded men and their bedding. The cradles should be in a berth by themselves, and each should be well cleated and secured to the decks, and sides of the ship. They should be so placed that you can easily go between them and tend to the dressings.

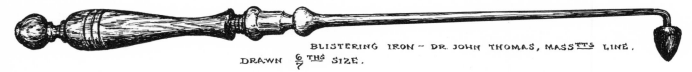

BLISTERING IRON - DR. JOHN THOMAS, MASS^{tts} LINE.
DRAWN $\frac{6}{7}$ THS SIZE.

THE PAY CRUNCH

Continental surgeons fought the high cost of living along with disease. The pay scale granted by Congress fell far short of that given to the line officers. Meanwhile, the value of the Continental currency decreased as steadily as the surgeons' subsistence costs increased. It took two years of petitioning before Congress gave some measure of relief. In 1778, the surgeons received sixty dollars a month and forty dollars for mates.

There the matter rested until 1781. The army officers had previously received half-pay for life upon retirement, and now the surgeons were awarded like benefits. As an added bonus, "equal" pay allowances were made to both medical and military branches. Welcomed as this overdue relief must have been, the ranks upon which the pay raises were based were relative. For example, the Director-General of the Medical Department held a rank of Brigadier-General, but received only the pay of a lieutenant colonel. Other officers, not including the lower status of mates, received a captain's pay.

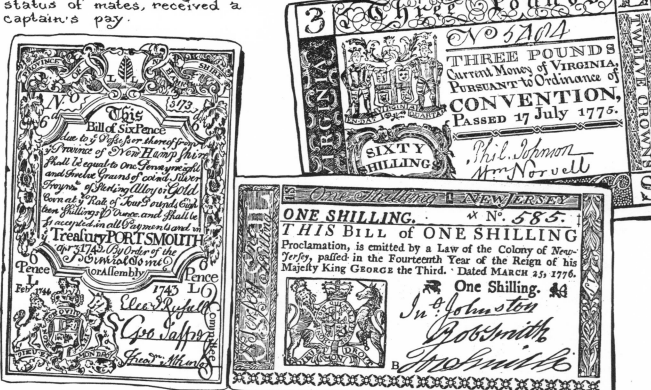

REVOLUTIONARY HIGHLIGHTS

All was not well between Mother England and her prized thirteen American colonies. By 1774 the voices of her free-thinking subjects had turned from "taxation only with parliamentary representation" to some form of self-government. No idle thoughts, these, for even now each colony was forming its own provincial congress ~ each with a voice to be heard clear across the Atlantic.

Insubordination could not be tolerated by the Crown. Since Massachusetts seemed to hold most of the troublemakers, Boston-based redcoats were soon marching through the surrounding towns to appropriate any and all militia military stores. The illegal Massachusetts Provincial Congress immediately set a Committee of Safety in motion to keep tabs on whatever mischief the British troops might be up to. Physician-surgeons were well represented among the Sons of Liberty.

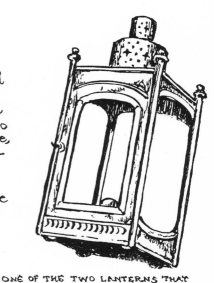

ONE OF THE TWO LANTERNS THAT HUNG IN OLD NORTH CHURCH.

JOIN OR DIE

REVERE ALSO A DENTIST?

Take Paul Revere for example. His talents were many and included the engraving of broadsides, seals and documents, cartoons lambasting those of Tory persuasion, and even a songbook. He was an expert silversmith, bellmaker, inventor, the first American to roll sheet copper ~ AND a respected dental surgeon.

His place in the allied medical arts was assured with his crafting of artificial teeth from ivory. Two such teeth were made and fitted for his good friend and high Son of Liberty, Dr. Joseph Warren. Revere's advertisement in the July 30, 1770 Boston Gazette Country Journal assured the reader that his tooth replacements were not only ornamental but also "of real use in Speaking and Eating." It seems that Revere was a jack of all trades and master of most.

THIRTYSIX-SHILLINGS.

Issued in defence of American Liberty.

Ense petit placidam sub Libertate Quietem.

Decmr. 7. 1775.

ENGRAVING BY REVERE IN 1775

DR. PRESCOTT'S RIDE INTO HISTORY

Paul Revere was once again galloping on the road to Lexington and Concord. Only two days earlier he'd been sent by Dr. Joseph Warren of the Committee of Safety to warn Concord that a British column might be marching to seize the militia stores of powder and weapons. This ride on the night of April 18, 1775 had added urgency, for not only were the British assembling for the anticipated raid, but they also hoped to snatch up the two rebel leaders, Sam Adams and John Hancock, as they slept the night in Lexington.

While Revere took one route, fellow alarm rider William Dawes

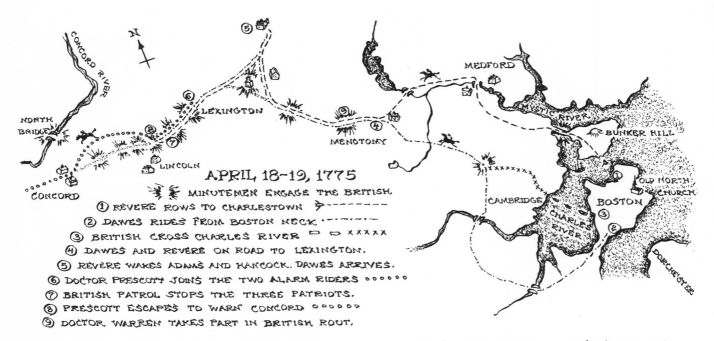

APRIL, 18-19, 1775

MINUTEMEN ENGAGE THE BRITISH

① REVERE ROWS TO CHARLESTOWN
② DAWES RIDES FROM BOSTON NECK
③ BRITISH CROSS CHARLES RIVER
④ DAWES AND REVERE ON ROAD TO LEXINGTON.
⑤ REVERE WAKES ADAMS AND HANCOCK. DAWES ARRIVES.
⑥ DOCTOR PRESCOTT JOINS THE TWO ALARM RIDERS
⑦ BRITISH PATROL STOPS THE THREE PATRIOTS.
⑧ PRESCOTT ESCAPES TO WARN CONCORD
⑨ DOCTOR WARREN TAKES PART IN BRITISH ROUT.

took another, should one be stopped by a mounted patrol. They met to awaken all of Lexington, then started on the last leg of the ride to Concord. The new day, the 19th, was but one hour along when Dr. Samuel Prescott fell in with the pair. This fellow Son of Liberty had been on a late house call of sorts, for he had been courting Lydia Mulliken. When they arrived at the still-lit Bull Tavern, Revere scouted the road ahead while Prescott and Dawes broke up a bit of sparking between Nathaniel Baker and Elizabeth Taylor. Baker was soon off to South Lincoln to alert the Minutemen~the name given to each towns' most active and adventuresome militiamen who could be called out at a minute's notice.

Revere was about 200 yards beyond the tavern when he caught sight of two figures partially outlined in the moonlight. In a moment they materialized into four mounted British officers, blocking the way with drawn pistols. G-d d--n you, stop! If you go another inch further, you are a dead man!" Prescott, who hadn't been far behind with Dawes, galloped up with the butt end of his whip turned and ready to do battle, but facing four pistol muzzles was a powerful argument against hasty heroics. The three patriots were forced to ride into an enclosed pasture for questioning.

Suddenly Dr. Prescott yelled "put on!" and spurred his horse for a jump over a low section of the stone wall. Two of the officers were soon after him, but the Concord doctor lost them in the blackness of a familiar ravine. While Revere was recaptured, Prescott made straight for the Town House alarm bell, sending its wakeup call clanging in the chill morning air. Tradition has it that Prescott continued his ride to alert the Minutemen of Acton and Stow.

ONE OF A PAIR OF SCOTTISH FLINTLOCK PISTOLS LOST AT LEXINGTON BY MAJOR PITCAIRN OF THE ROYAL MARINES. THE AMERICAN GENERAL PUTNAM USED THEM THROUGHOUT THE WAR.

The practice of medicine had long been a tradition in the Prescott family. Samuel's father, Dr. Abel, was the son and grandson of physicians. Samuel's older brothers were also doctors. Benjamin joined the Continental Army as a surgeon and later returned to his Concord practice. Abel Jr. carried the muster alarm to the nearby towns of Sudbury and Framingham, then returned for his musket to help hurry the retreating redcoated columns back to Boston. He recovered from a shoulder wound received in the action, only to die a short five months later of dysentery.

As for Samuel Prescott, he had made his last visit to Lydia Mulliken's home. The retreating British had torched the house and barn and burned them to the ground. We do know that Prescott served as surgeon with the Massachusetts troops in 1776 at Fort Ticonderoga. He then signed aboard a privateering ship, was captured at sea, and was thrown into a Halifax prison. There he died while Lydia remained in the area to await his return. Unaware of her lover's fate, she continued to hold out hope for eight years after the final Yorktown victory in 1781. Only then did she marry another and move to another town with her memories.

THE CANADIAN THREAT

Canada seemed much like a cannon ready for loading, with its muzzle pointed southward toward the rebellious New England colonies. Almost before any sort of Continental Army had taken shape, Washington ordered overland marches to Montreal and Quebec ~ perhaps to be joined by French Canadians of like mind. The Quebec attack would be led by flamboyant Colonel Benedict Arnold on what was probably the most imaginative and ambitious offensive of the war. According to the maps, the march to Quebec appeared to be little more than a stroll in the woods that would follow the cruise from Boston to Maine and a row up the Kennebec River in a fleet of bateaux. And so, in September 1775, some 1,100 colonial troops set off to face an unbelievable 350-mile nightmare of rapids, brutal portages, floods, drenching rains, ice and snow underfoot, hunger, and devastating illnesses.

Arnold's surgeon was strapping twenty-two-year old Isaac Senter, fresh from completing his apprenticeship. Dr. Senter jotted down the day-to-day happenings, and by the time they'd reached Norridgewock Falls, the rapids and portages had accounted for many wrecked bateaux and water-spoiled casks of fish, bread, and peas. Tainted food may well have caused the growing presence of dysentery and diarrhea among the troops. Of no help to their recovery was Senter's observation that "our fare was reduced to salt pork and flour."

By the middle of October, Dr. Senter had much to say about the Great Carrying Place. "The Army was now much fatigued, being obliged to carry all the bateaux, barrels of provisions, warlike stores, etc., over their backs [each bateau weighed 400 pounds and was portaged by four soldiers] through the most terrible piece of woods conceivable. Sometimes in the mud knee deep, then over ledgy hills, etc." Then "many of us are in a sad plight with the diarrhea. Our water was of the worst quality...No sooner had it got down, than it was puked up by many of the poor fellows." So many fell ill that "we now found it necessary to erect a building for the reception

QUEBEC

CHAUDIERE RIVER

MONTREAL

GREAT CARRYING PLACE

ANDROSCOGGIN RIVER

KENNEBEC RIVER

NORRIDGEWOCK FALLS

1775-1776
AMERICAN MARCH
TO QUEBEC

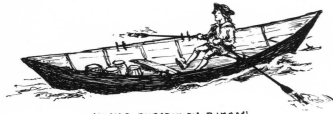

ARNOLD EXPEDITION BATEAU

of our sick."

A miscalculated supply of rations had placed the men on half rations by mid-October, and the doctor mentioned that one division found it necessary to eat their candles "by boiling them in water gruel." One division up and returned home just when a raw kind of courage was needed. The sick continued a retreat to Dr. Senter's makeshift hospital. By November 1 the doctor wrote that "our greatest luxuries now consisted in a little water, stiffened with flour in imitation of shoemaker's paste" that "instead of diarrhea, which tried our men most shockingly in the former part of our march, the reverse was now the complaint, which continued for many days." Finally ~ the next day in fact ~ 650 gaunt, ragged, and starving survivors of the march at last arrived at the Chaudiere River where there was a decent amount of food on the hoof.

ARNOLD'S PATRIOTIC LEG

Once on Canadian soil, the famine-proof veterans (as they called themselves) were in a position to join with Montgomery's victorious troops ~ already on their way from Montreal. The combined American army of about 1,000 volunteer soldiers would now face more than 1,200 well-entrenched veteran redcoats, British seamen and marines, as well as any handy British militia or Quebec gentry. Unfortunately, the French Canadians didn't join in a bid for freedom, but rather were content to remain on the sidelines and watch their old French and Indian War enemies shoot it out.

Drifting snows had already given the newcomers a taste of a northern winter. Laying siege to a snug enemy in such a deep freeze without adequate powder and heavy artillery had no chance for success. Time was running out, for the volunteer enlistments were nearly completed. And so it was that in the fury of an early morning blizzard on December 31, 1775 that the Americans launched a two-pronged attack on Quebec. Until fate stepped in, it did seem as though Canada would become the fourteenth member of the thirteen originals. But General Montgomery and his officers were killed by a single cannon blast while leading a lower town charge, and Arnold was leveled by a musket ball in the left leg. Leaderless, the assault sputtered and went out like a wet fuse.

American casualties, including a frustrated Arnold, made their way to a small hospital beyond the city. When a report came that the British might be advancing, Dr. Senter reported that "under these circumstances we entreated Colonel Arnold for his own safety be carried back into the country but to no purpose. He would neither be removed, nor suffer a man from the hospital to retreat. He ordered his pistols loaded, with a sword on his bed etc. We were now all soldiers, even the wounded in their beds were ordered a gun by their bedside." Fortunately the British did not pursue ~ and find they had a wounded tiger by the tail.

ST. LAWRENCE RIVER

MONTREAL

RICHELIEU RIVER

LAKE CHAMPLAIN

ARNOLD'S FLOTILLA STALLED BRITISH AT VALCOUR ISLAND

FORT TICONDEROGA

LAKE GEORGE

SARATOGA BATTLEFIELD

HUDSON RIVER

ALBANY

However, pursue they did by the fall of 1776 with an impressive squadron spearheading down Lake Champlain to ultimately cut the New England rebels off from their sister colonies. Somehow Arnold cobbled together enough timber that would float and enough cannon power to stall the drive until next year. When a combined British and German mercenary force returned to complete their Lake Champlain, Lake George, and Hudson River wedge they met a crushing defeat at the hands of the Continental Army at Saratoga.

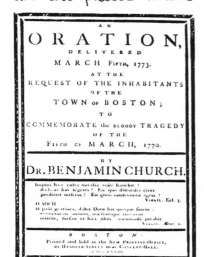

ARNOLD'S TWICE WOUNDED LEG ON AN UNMARKED MONUMENT AT THE SARATOGA BATTLE-FIELD WAS THE ONLY PART OF HIM WORTH CALLING AMERICAN.

Again Arnold, now wearing a general's braid, made his appearance leading a reckless but very successful charge to take several enemy redoubts. He received another musket ball in the same leg as the Quebec battle wound. But any admiration from his countrymen died with his later traitorous dealings with the enemy. His left leg was thereafter considered the only patriotic and worthwhile part of his anatomy.

UNMASKING ANOTHER TRAITOR

Well before the name Benedict Arnold became synonymous with betrayal, a like mind was working behind the scenes. For more than six months before the Lexington and Concord skirmishes, the British command had knowledge of the location and the amount of powder and armament stored at Concord. They knew that Sam Adams and John Hancock could be captured quite handily when the redcoats made their April 18 night march. And for well over a month the plans to fortify Bunker Hill were in enemy hands. "It was a common opinion," Paul Revere later recalled, "that there was a Traytor in the Provincial Congress, and that Gage was possessed of all their Secrets." At the time, British General Thomas Gage was Massachusetts' governor and also the British military commander in the colonies.

Revere had uneasy feelings about the highly regarded Dr. Benjamin Church of Boston. "He appeared to be a high Son of Liberty. He frequented all the places where they met, Was incouraged by all the leaders of the Sons of Liberty, and it appeared he was respected by them, though I knew that Dr. Warren had not the greatest affection for him." Hadn't he parodied some of the liberty songs in favor of the British, been seen in the company of British officers and even made an occasional visit to General Gage himself? But suspicions were blunted by his reasonable-enough answer that he did so to learn of any forthcoming enemy moves.

Church's credentials were the best ~ a Harvard graduate, outstanding surgeon, and unanimously elected director and chief physician of the first Continental Army hospital at Cambridge July 25, 1775. And so he continued to move freely about occupied Boston, at least until his coded letter was mistakenly left with a patriot in Newport, Rhode Island where a British fleet was based. The word of its translations swept through the colonies like wildfire. Ebenezer Huntington, a young Continental soldier who had left his studies at Yale to join the rebels two days after the Concord battle,

AN
ORATION,
DELIVERED
MARCH FIFTH, 1773.
AT THE
REQUEST OF THE INHABITANTS
OF THE
TOWN OF BOSTON;
TO
COMMEMORATE the BLOODY TRAGEDY
OF THE
FIFTH OF MARCH, 1770.

BY
DR. BENJAMIN CHURCH.

BOSTON:
Printed and Sold at the New Printing-Office,
in Hanover Street near Concert-Hall.

summed up the news in a letter to his brother.

...You will be much surprised to hear that our famous Doctor Church, that great pretended patriot, is now under a special guard of a captain and forty men for corrosponding with Gage and other of his hellish gang. The plot was discovered by his miss, who is now with child by him and he owns himself the father (for he has dismissed his wife). She was the bearer of some of his letters from this place (Roxbury) to Newport to Captain Wallace who hath the forwarding them to Boston. She left them with a man she supposed friendly to Doctor Church, but was mistaken; he having a curiosity to know the contents opened them, but they were wrote in characters so that he was not able to understand them, but guessing the contents, brought the letters and girl to General Washington, who after an examination and four hours under guard confessed she carried them from Doctor Church. His trial has not been yet, but suppose it will be ere long...

Church refused to decipher his coded letter, and so Washington turned its three pages over to three officers in his new army who were familiar with coded messages. All reached the same translation by using "frequency distribution." The most used letters in English in descending order generally are ETOANIRSHDL. The most numerous symbols or letters in Church's code, then, would be considered as E, the next most plentiful would represent T, and so on. Because the letters of J, K, Q, X, and Z are written so infrequently, Church simply used them without coding them. So much for his secret alphabet soup.

A SMALL SECTION OF PAGE 5, FROM CHURCH'S CRYPTOGRAM   JULY, 1775

The forty-four year old Doctor impressed few with his plea that he simply was inflating the patriots' numbers and capabilities to push the British into an advantageous peace. None the less, the once admired Church was judged guilty by court-martial on October 4, 1775. Such traitorous activity against one's country should have been punishable by death. However, when Congress adopted the Articles of War in June of that year, the penalty for dealing with the enemy was only thirty-nine lashes, two month's pay fine, or be drummed out of the army in disgrace. The option to stretch the rascal's neck with a rope was soon added~ but too late to apply to Church's case.

Dr. Church was confined to prison, but then given temporary parole because of his worsening asthma. On January 9, 1778, Church was ordered to leave the country. He was placed aboard the sloop Welcome bound for the island of Martinique on January 12, 1778. The vessel was lost with all hands. As for any question of Dr. Church being a misjudged patriot, years later the records and papers among General Thomas Gage's effects left no doubt that he was a dedicated spy in the pay of the British.

THE DOCTORS WARREN

Dr. Joseph Warren could serve as a role model for any young man apprenticing for the medical profession. At the age of fourteen he entered Harvard College, distinguished himself in his studies and apprenticed under a Boston physician. Tall and handsome, fair and blue-eyed, Dr. Warren was a catch by any measure ~ or so thought Elizabeth Hooton of Boston. She brought a handsome dowry to their marriage and later two sons and two daughters. Meanwhile the practice was booming, thanks to his growing reputation in Boston town.

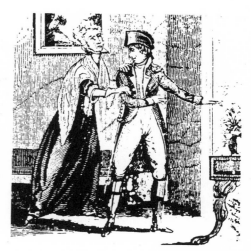

AFTER A MUSKET BALL CLIPPED A LOCK OF JOSEPH'S HAIR DURING THE BRITISH RETREAT, HIS MOTHER PLEADED WITH HIM NOT TO RISK HIS LIFE AGAIN.

John Adams chanced by one day for a smallpox vaccination, and Dr. Warren's life was never again the same. His respected patient spoke of America's servitude under an overbearing parliament, and the doctor was on his way to becoming a Son of Liberty. With his practice on hold, Dr. Warren became a spokesman and writer for a united front against the Crown's repressive acts. As chairman of the Committee of Safety and then President of the Provincial Congress, he dispatched Paul Revere to other colonial congresses as far away as Philadelphia. And when the British troops marched on Lexington and Concord, he took up his musket to hurry their retreat back to Boston.

More bloodshed was now inevitable, and on June 14, 1775 the Provincial Congress elected Warren a major general of the Massachusetts colonial forces. Meanwhile he had some worry about General Putnam's occupation of Bunker Hill, with but a scanty supply of gunpowder on hand. Still, by June 17 a beehive of activity had been started by the patriot troops ~ and under the very noses of the British military across the Charles River. Since his commission was not yet in hand, he refused command when offered it by Putnam. Instead, he reported to the Breed's Hill redoubt as a volunteer. When that first defense was about to be overrun, Warren received a fatal musket shot to the head while trying to rally the men.

Perhaps Captain John Chester, whose Connecticut troops covered the Breed's Hill withdrawal to the more elevated Bunker Hill, best expressed the sorrow felt by every American that day. "Good Dr. Warren, God rest his soul, I hope is safe in heaven! Had many of their officers the spirit and courage in their whole constitution that he had in his little finger, we had never retreated."

Warren's youngest brother John had only just completed his two-year medical apprenticeship with him in Boston. Upon learning of his brother's death at Breed's Hill, he gave up his medical practice and volunteered for service in the ranks. When Washington arrived in Cambridge in July 1775, the Medical Department of the Continental Army was organized. John was but twenty-two years old when he was appointed senior surgeon at the Cambridge military hospital. The following year he saw service at Long Island and then doctored the troops at Taunton and Princeton. After the war, he added considerable prestige to the young nation as professor of anatomy and surgery at Harvard Medical School when it opened in 1782. Among his list of credits was performing America's first abdominal operation and pioneering shoulder joint surgery.

The Warren brothers were ready to lay down their lives for a more democratic America. Perhaps Jefferson found inspiration from all such patriots when he penned the Declaration of Independence.

SIGNING THE DECLARATION

"We hold these truths to be self-evident, that all men are created equal, that they are endowed by their Creator with certain unalienable rights, that among these are life, liberty, and the pursuit of happiness." Jefferson's Declaration of Independence would be the cornerstone of the newly united states IF approved by the representatives of each colony in the Continental Congress. For some, the revolutionary concept of self-government was daunting. As for Torys and Great Britain itself, signing such a document was a treasonous act punishable by death.

According to two well-known legends, Ben Franklin's answer was "We must indeed hang together, or most assuredly we shall all hang separately." And John Hancock remarked after signing his name that extended nearly 5 inches, that it was large enough for John Bull to read without his glasses.

Fifty-six signers did cut the ties with Great Britain that July day in 1776. Briefly, there were four doctors who wrote their "John Hancocks." The famous Dr. Benjamin Rush was a Pennsylvania delegate and has been mentioned several places in these pages. Dr. Lyman Hall, one of the signers from Georgia was a transplanted New Englander and the earliest leader among Georgia's patriots. He urged that colony to send delegates to the Continental Congress over Loyalist objections. After the Revolution, he became Governor of the state and set aside a grant of land for Georgia's first college.

The remaining two physician-surgeons hailed from New Hampshire. Dr. Matthew Thornton served with the New Hampshire troops in the 1746 Louisburg expedition and later as a colonel in the militia and was president of the New Hampshire Provincial Congress and chairman of the Committee of Safety. Dr. Joseph Bartlett was also a colonel in the militia, and in August 1777 he attended to the wounded from the Battle of Bennington. He continued to practice medicine after the war in addition to holding a seat on the Supreme Court bench, and still found time to charter the New Hampshire Medical Society in 1791.

Of interest is the list of medicines purchased by Bartlett in 1765~ all rather typical of many medicines used in those revolutionary times.

3¾ oz. Sp. Lavand	Spirits of Lavender for aromatic stimulant, tonic, and perfume
4¼ oz. Sal Ammon	Salts of Ammonia for purging the intestine
1¼ oz Ol. Anisi	Oil of Anise to relieve the passage of wind
1 oz. Rad Rhis	Root of Sumac for urinary incontinence
4 oz. Rad Salopii	Root of a Near East orchid for softening the stools
4 oz. G. Cambog	Gum of an East Indian tree for a powerful cathartic and expulsion of tapeworms
2 oz Pul. Ipecacuanh	Pulverized ipecac root from South America used in large doses as an emetic and smaller amounts as a diaphoretic and expectorant

½ lb. Flor Sulph — Flowers of sulfur (a fancy term meaning purified sulfur powder) used as a laxative, joint pain, and a scabies specific

½ lb. G. Aloes Shepert — Gum Aloes dried from the mucilaginous sap of the aloe plants for the Caribbean and Africa. Uses include an intestinal cathartic

It would seem that much of Dr. Bartlett's practice involved ridding the intestines of whatever irritant might be causing "excitability."

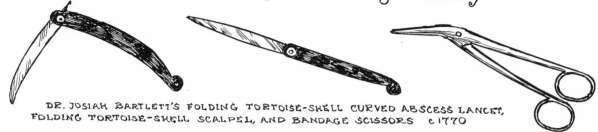

DR. JOSIAH BARTLETT'S FOLDING TORTOISE-SHELL CURVED ABSCESS LANCET, FOLDING TORTOISE-SHELL SCALPEL, AND BANDAGE SCISSORS c.1770

HEAL WITHOUT HARM

It was Voltaire who observed that "a physician is one who pours drugs of which he knows little into a body of which he knows less." Actually, there were but three medicines in the eighteenth-century doctor's bag of tricks that could honestly be called curative.

1. "Fever-bark" had long been used by the Peruvian Indians as a specific for recurrent chills followed by high fever — otherwise known as malaria. The dried-and-powdered bark of this South American tree yielded quinine. This medicine worked by destroying malarial parasites, which are spread by the anopheles mosquito bite and use red blood cells for their hosts. Once brought back to the old world, physicians used the fever-bark for any illness with a fever.

Since the onset of malarial symptoms often followed exposure to warm, damp, and swampy areas, it seemed reasonable in those days to assume that bad air, or "mal-area," was the cause.

2. Vitamin C (ascorbic acid), plentiful in citrus fruits, was the cure for scurvy. The disease was the scourge of sailors on long sea voyages. James Lind, a Scottish naval surgeon aboard the H.M.S. Salisbury in 1747, was shocked to find almost a fourth of the crew had scurvy and many became fatalities. His Treatise of the Scurvy, published in 1753, called for a diet of lemon juice to be added to the sailors' daily rations. Almost overnight the symptoms of weakness; weight loss; aches and pains; small hemorrhages; spongy, bleeding gums; loosening of the teeth; and poor wound healing disappeared with the ingestion of lemon juice.

Unfortunately, the British Admiralty fumbled this gift of good health to its seamen. It wasn't until one year after Dr. Lind's death in 1795 that the lemon juice became the official shipboard cure. With a cure as simple as that, Jack Tar could reasonably be called a Limey.

3. The foxglove plant had long delighted English gardeners ~ and after 1785 patients with weak hearts would also be singing its praises. That was the year that Dr. William Withering published his Account of the Foxglove ~ a surprise to his medical colleagues. Botany had been his least favored course as a student.

FOXGLOVE

73

However, a patient of his, Miss Helena Cooke, soon changed all that. The young doctor fell in love with Miss Cooke and eventually married her. He then found botany tolerable indeed through his wife's talented drawings and paintings of flowers and plants.

Dr. Withering knew that foxglove had been used for centuries by herbalists for a hodge-podge of reasons. His curiosity led him into nine years of experimentation of its active ingredient, digitalis. He found the drug-containing leaves should be harvested and powdered just before the plant flowered. The remarkable discovery was able to strengthen a weak heart by contracting its muscles to give a strong and efficient output at a slower rate. In a day when more medicine might be considered better, Withering gave the specifics for a sufficient primary dose of digitoxin and a carefully regulated daily amount to prevent toxicity.

APOTHECARY FIRSTS

The Lexington and Concord battles had given the world notice of America's determination to live free or die. The Massachusetts Committee of Safety meanwhile had to provide for any patriots who might join the sick, wounded or disabled lists. On April 30, 1775, a promising young Boston apothecary, Andrew Craigie, was appointed the first Massachusetts Commissary of Medical Stores. The lack of the colonial medical supplies was obvious when he assisted physicians at the Battle of Bunker Hill.

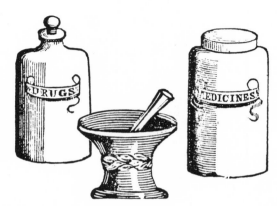

When in July 1775 the Continental Congress created the position of Apothecary General for each Army hospital, Craigie was the first man appointed. Two years later, he advanced to lieutenant colonel while continuing "to receive, prepare, and deliver medicines and other articles of his department to the hospitals and army." A year later he had suggested and established the first pharmaceutical laboratory at Carlisle, Pennsylvania, where quality medicines could be made in quantity. During that time he likely had a hand in producing the first American Pharmacopoeia. Craigie's service as Apothecary General on the Continental Army staff throughout the conflict helped to establish America's pharmaceutical standards.

A VALLEY FORGE IMPRESSION

The warm glow of the Saratoga victory was needed to cheer the dreary 1777~1778 wintering at Valley Forge. Dr. Albigence Waldo, the twenty-seven-year-old surgeon of the First Connecticut Infantry, wrote this tongue-in-cheek description of camp life in his diary.

"December 21. Preparations made for huts. Provisions scarce. Sent a letter to my wife. Heartily wish myself at home. My skin and eyes are almost spoiled with continual smoke. A general cry through the camp this evening among the soldiers, 'No meat! No meat!' The distant vales echoed back the melancholy sound, 'No meat! No meat!'

'What have you for your dinners, boys?'

'Nothing but fire cake and water, sir.'

At night, 'Gentlemen, the supper is ready.'

'What is your supper, lads?'

'Fire cake and water, sir.'

Very poor beef has been drawn in our camp the greater part of this season. A butcher, bringing a quarter of this kind of beef into camp one day, had white buttons on the knees of his breeches. A soldier cries out, "There, there, Tom, is some more of your fat beef. By my soul, I can see the butcher's breeches buttons through it.""

It almost seemed that Thomas Paine's _The American Crisis_ had Valley Forge in mind when he wrote:

"These are the times that try men's souls: The summer soldier and the sunshine patriot will, in this crisis, shrink from the service of his country; but he that stands it NOW deserves the love and thanks of man and woman. Tyranny, like Hell, is not easily conquered. Yet we have this consolation with us, that the harder the conflict, the more glorious the triumph."

And so it was that British troops would be facing an inspired American army of disciplined veterans, able to execute commands with a precision that gave great credit to their drillmaster, Baron von Steuben.

THE PERKINS TRACTOR CURE

The lively mind of Ben Franklin had produced his _Experiments in Electricity_ in 1753, and an attempt to stimulate the muscles of paralysis victims was a logical next step. Although Franklin signed off such efforts as failures, it was rumored that this extraordinary man could now cure dropsy and blindness. In 1786, the public interest was sparked when Luigi Galvani discovered what he called "animal electricity." Legs of freshly killed frogs, hung on a copper hook, began violent muscle contractions when they touched an iron support. Actually, as Volta later proved, it was the contact between two unlike metals that produced the current. Wags may have called Galvani "the Frog's Dancing Master," but the believers in electricity's curative powers were primed for the next discovery.

Dr. Elisha Perkins now appeared on center stage with his famous metallic tractors. The Connecticut doctor was no humbug, for he was a student at Yale and apprenticed to his highly regarded physician father. But it was during some of his surgical operations that he found the patient's muscles contracted when touched by his metallic instruments. It was then that his brainchild, "Perkin's Patent Tractors"
was born.

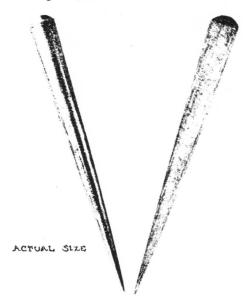

ACTUAL SIZE

PERKINS PATENT TRACTORS

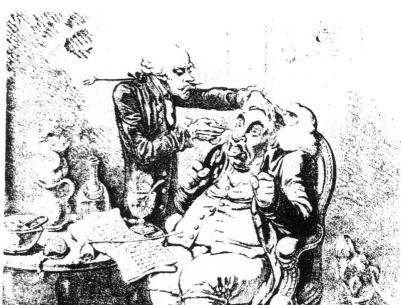

METALLIC TRACTORS ENGRAVING BY W. HUMPREY, LONDON 1801

Actually the tractors were nothing more than a brass and an iron awl that he made in a small home furnace. Each was about 3 inches long, half-rounded along one side with one end rounded and the other pointed. They were called "tractors" because they were alternately drawn or stroked over the affected part of the patient's anatomy.

Although his medical colleagues took a dim view of such quackery ~ the Connecticut Medical Society expelled him in 1796 ~ his electrical cure-alls sold like hotcakes here and in England. It was even said that George Washington had his own pair of curative tractors. Finally a London physician with two disguised wooden tractors duplicated Perkins "miracles," debunking the so-called cure. An expectant and optimistic mind is often the real curative power behind any treatment, then and now.

MYSTERIES OF THE MIND

It was a common eighteenth century belief that mental stress ~ fear, despair, jealousy, frustration, and depression ~ could bring one to the brink of lunacy. Heaven knows this host of emotions was in great plenty among both loyalists and rebels during those trying Revolutionary War days. Medical theory dictated that the excessive nerve stimulation could cause mental as well as physical illness. Blood vessels would be thrown into spasms and the congestion of blood that followed was bound to befuddle the mind. Dr. Benjamin Rush had an answer. The patient should have a massive bloodletting to reduce that congestion and any scrambled brain would be relieved in the semiconscious state that followed.

Drastic therapy indeed ~ so much so that Dr. Rush's compassion for these unfortunates and his other asylum reforms might be overlooked.

RUSH'S
TRANQUILIZING CHAIR

"Treatment" until then might have been little more than ice to the head and hot water to the feet to draw blood away from the head or opium to quiet maniacal ravings. Rush introduced a more humane approach with an early form of occupational therapy by providing spinning wheels and wool for the patients of Pennsylvania Hospital. There would be no chains and excessive restraints in cells that would now be kept clean, dry, and airy. Latrines and bathing facilities would be handy and a central corridor was built for patient exercises.

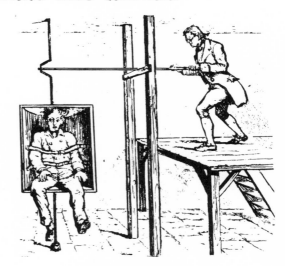

RUSH'S GYRATING CHAIR

In his effort to treat insanity by reducing or eliminating its causes, he pioneered such devices as the tranquilizing chair and the gyrating chair. And because of his innovative efforts, Dr. Rush is regarded as the founder of American psychiatry.

THE MADNESS OF KING GEORGE III

It was a heavy-handed parliament and not its king that decreed that its American subjects could be taxed without representation. Colonial discontent smoldered with each new taxation scheme until a bid for self-government seemed the only solution. This, of course, was

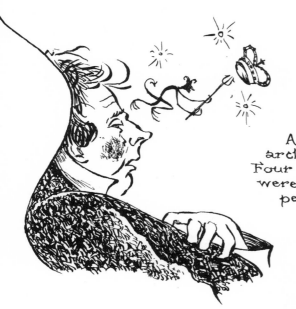

considered treason, and now King George must bring his authority to bear and preserve the Empire at all costs. The King was often obstinate and tactless when making royal decisions and his frustrations may have hurried him on a course to self-destruction. It was just five years after America won its independence that the monarch suffered his first mental breakdown. Four more episodes that bordered on madness were his lot until a full-blown nine-year period of insanity ended in his death in 1820.

Recently several medical detectives have offered the possibility that King George had an inherited illness. Their suspect is porphyria (Greek *porfura* meaning "purple"). Porphyrin is a vital part of all protoplasm and is the basic structure of hemoglobin. An inherited excess can flood the body and produce irritability, anxiety, confusion, and restlessness. More severe symptoms include convulsions, delirium, hallucinations and psychosis. As for the "purple" name, urine can turn that color when exposed to light. And as for King George III, we'll never really know the truth about his affliction.

AND IN CONCLUSION ~ DIVIDED SPECTACLES

Parliament's short-sighted views of the American colonies couldn't be corrected by Ben Franklin's spectacle invention in 1784. He'd found it a bother to substitute his far vision spectacles for a pair with near vision lenses each time he'd read or do close-up work. Franklin solved his problem~ and ours as well~ by placing half of a convex lens into the upper part of each eyerim frame. Far vision light rays would then converge to form a clear image instead of a blurred impression focused behind the retina. Then a half of a concave lens was positioned in each lower eyerim frame space. Near vision light rays would then be spread out to focus on the retina instead of falling short of the mark. Franklin's "divided spectacles" or "bifocals" still help to make aging eyesight young again.

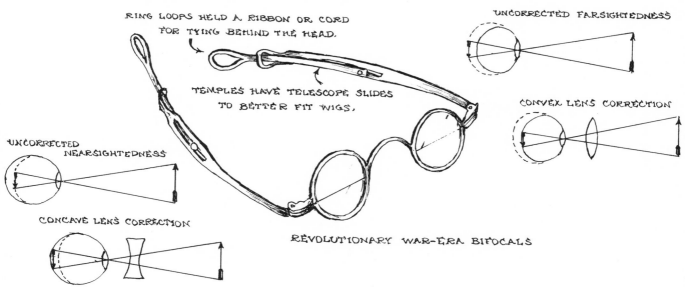

RING LOOPS HELD A RIBBON OR CORD FOR TYING BEHIND THE HEAD.

TEMPLES HAVE TELESCOPE SLIDES TO BETTER FIT WIGS.

UNCORRECTED FARSIGHTEDNESS

CONVEX LENS CORRECTION

UNCORRECTED NEARSIGHTEDNESS

CONCAVE LENS CORRECTION

REVOLUTIONARY WAR-ERA BIFOCALS

77

AND FINALLY~ The home grown American physician-surgeons were independent, outspoken, often cantankerous, of varied abilities and education~ and fiercely patriotic. These were the men who faced the medical crisis in Washington's army. There were no guidelines and no formulas, no supplies and no organization~ and mighty little support from Congress. Yet somehow the Hospital ~ the Medical Department~ made trial-and-error progress toward providing creditable care for their sick and wounded. Indeed, such medical giants as Morgan, Rush, Tilton, and Jones gave their new country some solid advances in efficiency, sanitation, hospital care, and surgical skills. American medicine had suddenly come of age. As with their country, they were no longer dutiful stepchildren under European dominance.

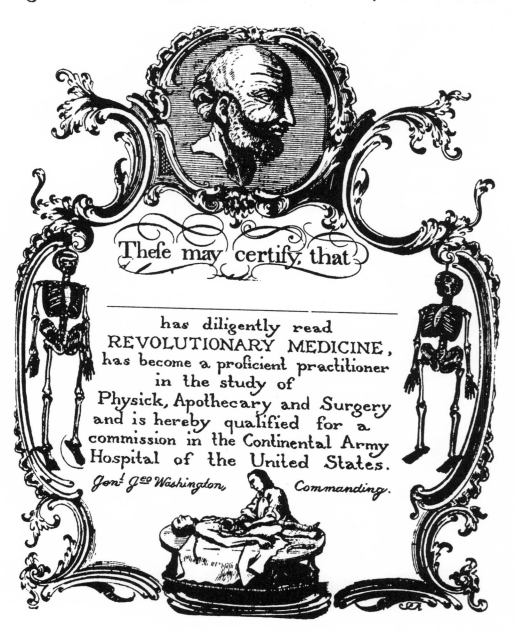

These may certify that

_____

has diligently read
REVOLUTIONARY MEDICINE,
has become a proficient practitioner
in the study of
Physick, Apothecary and Surgery
and is hereby qualified for a
commission in the Continental Army
Hospital of the United States.

Gen! Geo Washington,   *Commanding.*

References

Alexander, Franz G., M.D., and Selesnick, Sheldon T. *The History of Psychiatry.* New York: Harper & Row, Publishers 1966.

Beardsley, Ebenezer, M.D. *History of a Dysentery in the 22nd Regiment of the late Continental Army.* Proceedings of the New Haven County Medical Society for 1788.

Bettman, Otto L. *History of Medicine,* Second Printing, Springfield, Illinois: Charles C. Thomas, Publisher 1956.

Blair, Patrick, M.D., F.R.S. *Miscellaneous Observations In the Practise of Physick, Anatomy, and Surgery.* London: Printed for William Mears at the Lamb Without Temple-Bar, 1718.

Brown, John, M.D. *The Elements of Medicine; or: A Translation of the Elementa Medicinae Brunonis A New Addition.* Philadelphia: Printed by T. Dobson, At The Stonehouse, No. 41, Second-Street. MDCCXC.

Buchan, William, M.D. *Domestic Medicine; or the Family Physician; Being an Attempt to Render the Medical Art more generally useful by shewing people what is in their own power both with respect to the Prevention and Cure of Diseases.* The Second American Edition with considerable additions by the author. Philadelphia: Robert Bell, 1775.

Butterfield, L.H., ed. *The Letters of Benjamin Rush.* 2 vols. Princeton University Press, 1951.

Clarke, Herbert, *The Apothecary in Eighteenth-Century Williamsburg; being an account of his medical and chirurgical services as well as of his trade practices as a chemist.* Williamsburg, Va.: Colonial Williamsburg, 1965.

Commager, Henry Steele, and Morris, Richard B. *The Spirit of "Seventy-Six."* Indianapolis: Bobbs-Merrill, 1958.

Corcoran, A.C., M.D. *A Mirror Up To Medicine.* Philadelphia, New York & Montreal: J.B. Lippincott Co., 1961.

Corner, George W., ed. *The Autobiography of Benjamin Rush, His "Travels Through Life" together with his Commonplace Book for 1798-1813.* Published for the American Philosophical Society by Princeton University Press, 1948.

Cullen, William, M.D. *Lectures on the Malaria Medica, as delivered by William Cullen, M.D., Professor of Medicine in the University of Edinburgh, Now Published by Permission of the Author, and with many Corrections from the Collation of different manuscripts by the Editors.* Philadelphia: Robert Bell, 1775.

D'Amato, Cintio, "Medical Life in the Eighteenth Century: On Making Incisions in the Veins of the Hands." In *Source Book of Medical History,* compiled with notes by Logan Clendining, M.D., pp. 285-287. New York: Dover Publications Inc., Henry Schuman, N.D.

Dimsdale, Thomas. *Present Method of Innoculating for the Small-pox.* Philadelphia: 1771.

Duffy, John. *Epidemics in Colonial America.* Port Washington, N.Y.: Kennikat Press, 1972.

Garrison, Fielding H., M.D. *An Introduction to the History of Medicine,* Third Edition, Revised and Enlarged, Philadelphia and London: N.B. Saunders Company, 1924.

Gill, Harold B. *The Apothecary in Colonial Virginia.* Charlottesville, Va.: University Press of Virginia, 1972.

Goler, Robert I., Curator of Collections "The Healing Arts In Early America"(Booklet), New York City: Fraunces Tavern Museum, 1985.

Goodman, Nathan G. *Benjamin Rush, Physician and Citizen.* Philadelphia: University of Pennsylvania Press, 1934.

"Great Moments in Pharmacy" (Booklet). Parke, Davis & Co. Stories by George A. Bender, Paintings by Robert A. Thom. Detroit: Northwood Institute Press, 1966.

Hooper, R. *Compendious Medical Dictionary.* Boston: 1801.

Hume, Edgar Erskine. *Victories of Army Medicine.* Philadelphia, London and Montreal: J.B. Lippincott Co., 1943.

Jones, John, M.D. *Plain, Concise, and Practical Remarks on the Treatment of Wounds and Fractures; To which is added, an Appendix, On Camp and Military Hospitals.* Philadelphia: Robert Bell, in Third Street, MDCCLXXVI.

Knight, Nancy "Pain and its Relief" (Booklet). An Exhibition of the National Museum of American History, Smithsonian Institution, Washington, D.C.: 1983, 1986.

La Wall, Charles H., PhM., Phar.D., Sc.D., F.R.S.A. *Four Thousand Years of Pharmacy,* pp. 262-436. Philadelphia and London: J.B. Lippincott Co., 1927.

Malone, Dumas. *The Story of the Declaration of Independence.* New York: Oxford University Press, 1954.

Margotta, Roberto. *The Story of Medicine.* New York: Golden Press, 1967, 1968.

Matthews, Leslie G. *Antiques of the Pharmacy.* London: Bell & Sons, 1971.

Medicine in Colonial Massachusetts 1620-1820. A Conference Held 25 & 26 May 1978 by The Colonial Society of Massachusetts, Boston: The Colonial Society of Massachusetts, Distributed by the University Press of Virginia, 1980.

Mevers, Frank C., Editors *The Papers of Josiah Bartlett.* Published for the New Hampshire Historical Society by the University

Press of New England, Hanover, New Hampshire, 1979.

Moore, John. *Medical Sketches: in Two Parts.* Providence: 1794.

Morgan, John, M.D. F.R.S. *A Vindication of His Public Character In the Station of Director-General of the Military Hospitals, and Physician-In-Chief to the American Army, Anno, 1776.* Boston: Powers and Willis, MDCCLXXVII.

Morgan, John, M.D., F.R.S., & Co. Director-General of the Hospitals, and Physician-In-Chief of the American Army. *A Recommendation of Inoculation, according to Baron Dimsdale's method.* Boston: J. Gill, in Queen-Street, MDCCLXXVI.

Mulliken, John Butter, M.D. "Prescott's People," pages 10-12. Physician East, Journal of Physicians' Interest, July 1981.

Murray, Eleanor M. "The Medical Department of the Revolution." *The Bulletin of the Fort Ticonderoga Museum* VII:3 (Jan. 1949) pp. 83-109.

Packard, Francis R., M.D. *History of Medicine in the United States,* vol. 1. New York: Paul B. Hoeber, Inc., 1931.

Parsons, Usher, M.D. *Sailor's Physician, Exhibiting the Symptoms, Causes and Treatment of Diseases Incident to Seamen and Passengers in Merchant Vessels with Directions for Preserving Their Health in Sickly Climates: Intended to Afford Medical Advice to Such Persons While at Sea where A Physician Cannot be Consulted.* Cambridge: Hilliard and Metcalf, 1820.

Paul Revere's Three Accounts of His Famous Ride with an Introduction by Edmund S. Morgan. A Revolutionary War Bicentennial Commission and Massachusetts Historical Society Publication, Boston: 1967.

Pendleton, James, Jun. of Virg., Member of the Philadelphia Medical and American L'inneal Society. *An essay on the Most Fundamental Principals in the Science of Medicine.* Washington: Samuel Harrison Smith, 1803.

Peterson, Michael L. The Church Cryptogram: To Catch A Tory Spy. p. 34–43. "American History Illustrated" November/December, Historical Times, Gettysburg, Pennsylvania.

Potts, Jonathan, M.D. Large collection of original manuscripts, furlough papers, cash accounts, payments and letters pertaining to medicine in the Revolution. Fort Ticonderoga Museum Library, Ticonderoga, NY.

Quincy, John. *Pharmacopoeia Officinalis & Extemporanea: A Complete English Dispensatory, in Two Parts, Theoretic and Practical.* London: 1761.

Ranby, John, Esq., Surgeon General to the British Army. *The Diseases Incident to Armies, with the Method of Cure.* Translated from the Original of Baron Van Swieten, Physicians to their Imperial Magesties. To which are added; To Be Observed by the Sea Surgeons in Engagements, Also, Preventatives of the Scurvy at Sea. By William Northcote, Surgeon, Many Years in the Sea-Service. Published for the use of Military, and Naval Surgeons in America. Philadelphia: Printed. Boston: Reprinted by E. Draper, for J. Douglass McDougall opposite the Old-South Meeting-House, MDCCLXXVII.

Riznik, Barnes. *Medicine in New England, 1790-1840.* Sturbridge, Mass.: Old Sturbridge Village, 1965.

Riznik, Barnes. *Rules for Regulation of the Navy of the United Colonies of North-America.* Philadelphia: William and Thomas Bradford, 1775.

Rush, Benjamin. M.D. *Medicine Inquiries and Observations.* 4 vols. 3d ed. Philadelphia: 1809.

Rush, Benjamin, M.D. *To the Officers in the Army of the United American States: Directions for Preserving the Health of Soldiers.* Published by Order of Board of War, 1777.

Singer, Charles, and Underwood, E. Ashworth. *A Short History of Medicine.* 2d ed. pp. 181-191. New York and Oxford: Oxford University Press, 1962.

Stoler, Margaret. Benjamin Church, Son of Liberty, Tory Spy p. 28–35. "American History Illustrated" November/December 1989, Historical Times, Gettysburg, Pennsylvania.

Stubbs, S.G. Blaxland, and Bligh, E.W. *Sixty Centuries of Health And Physick.* pp. 168-219. Great Britain: Paul B. Hoeber, Inc., New York, MCMXXI.

Thacher, James, M.D. *American Medical Biography, or Memoirs of Eminent Physicians Who Have Flourished in America.* First published in 1828. New York: Milford House, Inc., MCMLXVII.

Thacher, James, M.D. *Military Journal of the American Revolution To Which Has Been Added The Life of Washington.* Hartford, Conn.: Hurlbert, Williams & Company, 1862.

Tilton, Dr. James. *Economic Observations on Military Hospitals and the Prevention of Diseases Incident to an Army.* Wilmington: 1813.

Thompson, C.J.S., M.B.E. *The Mystery and Art of The Apothecary.* pp. 250-282. J.B. Lippincott Co., 1929.

Toner, J.M., M.D. *The Medical Men of The Revolution.* Philadelphia: Collins, Printer, 705 Jayne Street, 1876.

Viets, Henry R. M.D. *A Brief History of Medicine in Massachusetts.* pp. 53-118. Cambridge: Houghton, Mifflin Co., The Riverside Press, 1930.

Wood, George B., M.D. *Treatise of the Practice of Medicine* Fifth Edition, Vol II Philadelphia: J.B. Lippincott and Co. 1858.

Wood, George B., M.D., and Bache, Franklin, M.D. *The Dispensatory of the United States of America* 8th ed. Carefully Revised. Philadelphia: Grigg, Elliot, and Co., 1849.

Where Illustrated Relics May Be Found

page

3   Dr. Shippen's anatomical drawings, Pennsylvania Hospital, Philadelphia, Pa.

4   Captain Phillips' eye stone, Fort Ticonderoga, Ticonderoga, New York.

8   Pierre Lyonet's microscope for Microdissection Med. Museum of Armed Forces—Institute of Pathology, Washington, D.C.

9   Wooden stethoscope, 1816-1819, Medical Museum of Armed Forces, etc.

10   Thomas Jefferson's lancet, Monticello, Virginia. Many-bladed fleam, Author's Collection. Dr. Richard Osborne's folding lancet, Washington's Headquarters Newburg, New York.

11   Pewter bleeding bowl, Hugh Mercer's Apothecary Shop, Fredericksburg, Virginia. Pewter syringe, Fort Ticonderoga, New York.

12   Glass & clay medicine bottles, wooden pill box, tortoise shell tweezers, Fort Ticonderoga, New York.

16   Dr. Benjamin Rush's medicine chest, from 1965 exhibition, "The Art of Philadelphia Medicine," Philadelphia Museum of Art, Philadelphia, Pa. Captain James Moore's Gravestone—Four miles upstream from Washington's Crossing to Trenton, New Jersey on Christmas Eve, 1776.

17   Eighteenth century crutch, Fort Ticonderoga, New York.

18   Molded horn drinking cup, Washington's Headquarters, Newburg, New York. Rifleman's noggin, Northampton Historical Society, Northampton, Mass.

19   Water bottle, Bennington Museum, Bennington, Vermont. Interlocking wooden strap canteen and bent strip canteen, Author's Collection. Tin canteen, Fort Ticonderoga, New York. Drowning exhibit—Museum of Science and Industry, Chicago, Ill. Destroyed by fire in 1963.

20   Interior view, Dr. Hugh Mercer's Apothecary Shop, Fredericksburg, Virginia.

21   Carboy, Dr. Hugh Mercer's Apothecary Shop. Ointment and drug jars, National Museum of History and Technology of the Smithsonian Institution, Washington, D.C.

22   Medicine bottle, Fort Ticonderoga, New York. Delft syrup and medicine jars, National Museum of History and Technology, etc.

23   Crude medicinals, National Museum of History and Technology, etc.

24   Crude medicinals, National Museum of History and Technology, etc.

24   General Henry Knox's mortar and pestle, National Museum of History and Technology, etc.

25   Brass mortar and pestle, National Museum of History and Technology, etc.

26   Ceramic pill tile, Dr. Hugh Mercer's Apothecary Shop, etc. Gas collectors, National Museum of History and Technology, etc.

29   Dr. Joshua Fisher's medicine chest, Beverly Historical Society, Beverly, Mass.

30   John O'Neil's razor and honing stone, Washington's Headquarters, Newburg, New York.

31   Eighteenth century scissors, Fort Ticonderoga, New York.

     Dr. John Thomas' surgical scissors and bullet forceps, Washington's Headquarters, Newburg, New York.

32   Screw tourniquet, Morristown National Historical Park, Morristown, N.J. Dr. Solomon Drowne's probes, tenaculum and scalpel, Fort Ticonderoga, New York. Crooked needle, Fort Ticonderoga, New York. Retractor and curved amputation knife, Medical Museum of Armed Forces, Institute, etc. Amputation saw and straight amputation knife, Medical Museum of Armed Forces Institute, etc.

33   Forceps, Medical Museum of Armed Forces Institute, etc.

36   Amputation saw, National Museum of History and Technology, etc.

38   Trepanning instrument, Medical Museum of Armed Forces Institute, etc.

40   Tooth extractor, Author's Collection. Washington's first dentures, New York Academy of Medicine, New York, N.Y. Washington's second dentures, National Museum of History and Technology, etc.

44   Pewter thunder jug, Mariners Museum, Newport News, Virginia.

45   Wigwam construction, from contemporary print, New York Historical Society, New York, N.Y.

46   Log hospital plan, military, from Dr. James Tilton's Economical Observations.

47   "Markee," similar to Washington's marquis, National Museum of History and Technology, etc.

48   Connecticut regimental buttons, Picture Book of the Continental Soldier, Stackpole, 1969.

49   Solomon Moore's shaving set, Fort Ticonderoga, New York.

50   British brass comb, New York Historical Society, New York, New York.

51   Soldier's shoe, Picture Book of the Continental Soldier, Stackpole, 1969.

52   Washington's folding camp bed, Mount Vernon Collection, Mount Vernon, Virginia.

53   Washington's toilet set, Mount Vernon Collection, Mount Vernon, Virginia.

54   Colonel Frederick Baume's camp stove, Bennington Museum, Bennington, Vermont. Cast iron kettle, Bennington Museum, Bennington, Vermont. Camp stove, Author's Collection. Washington's cooking pot, National Museum of History and Technology, etc. Brass tent cooking pot, Fort Ticonderoga, New York.

55   Washington's liquor case, Mount Vernon Collection, Mount Vernon, Virginia. Glassware, liquor bottles, New York Historical Society, New York, New York.

56   Sun design from Rising Sun Tavern, built 1760, Fredericksburg, Virginia—a popular meeting place for George Washington, Hugh Mercer, Thomas Jefferson, George Mason, Patrick Henry, John Marshall and the Lees of Virginia.

57   Catchpenny prints from the Eighteenth Century, originally published by Bowles & Carver. Reprinted by Dover Press. Woodcut from Newburyport, Massachusetts broadside.

58   Eighteenth century anchor, Picture Book of the

Revolution's Privateers, Stackpole, 1973.

60 Dried potatoes, Peabody Maritime Museum, Salem, Mass.

61 Hard Tack, Peabody Maritime Museum, Salem, Mass. Ivory medicine dropper, Washington's Headquarters, Newburg, N.Y.

64 Blistering iron, Washington's Headquarters, Newburg, N.Y.

65 Old North Church lantern, Concord Atheneum, Concord, Mass.

69 Medicine scales, Washington's Headquarters, Newburg, N.Y.

70 Certificate—engraved border by Paul Revere for Certificate of Attendance, Dr. Warren's lectures in Boston, 1782.

Index

Italicized words and numbers indicate illustrations.

A

Adams, John, 71
    anatomical notes, 3
Adams, Sam, 65, 69
additives, 25
adhesive plaster, 33
Aedes Aegypti, 15
ague, 12
air, in camp, 52
Albany, New York, hospital at, 38
Alchemy symbols
    antimony, 24
    borax, 24
    ginger, 24
    honey, 24
    mercury, 24
    sugar, 24
    sulphur, 24
    verdigris, 24
    vinegar, 24
    wine spirits, 24
alcohol, 12, 13
alum, 15
aloe gum, 73
ambulance precursors, 28
American Crises, The, 75
American Plague, 15
ammonia, 72
amputation, 34, 36
amputation knives, 32
amputation, leg, 36
amputation, saw, 32, 36
Anatomy, 1, 2
    anatomical drawings, 3
    comments by John Adams, 3
    course described, 3
    models, Dr. Chovet's, 3
    "Resurrectionists," 2, 3
anatomy of a ship, 58
anchor, eighteenth century, 58
Angina Suffocativa, 14
Angina Ulcusculosa, 14
anise, 13
antiarthritics, 11
antidysentery medications, 11
antimony symbol, 24
antipyretics, 12
anodynes, 11, 13, 17
aorta, wounds of, 30
Apothecary, Army, 20
Apothecary, Dr. Hugh Mercer's, 11
Apothecary, Hospital
    commission, 22
Apothecary shops, 21
Apothecary signs, 21
Apprentice system, 1

Anatomy, 2, 3
    Certificate of Proficiency, 1
    examinations to practice, 4
    in Army, 20
    in large cities, 2
    lectures, 2
    qualifications for, 1
    Osteology, description of, 2
    tasks, 2
    teacher-physicians, 1
    time required, 1
    subjects learned, 1
Army Regulations, Steuben's, 47
Army Surgeon at work, 27
Arnold, Benedict, 67–69
ascorpic acid, 73
atropine, 23

B

bandage, eighteen tail, 35
bandage, compress, 35
bandaging, 2
barber, regimental, 49
Barbadoes Distemper, 15
"Bark," 11, 12, 16
barley water, 12
barrels, meat, 53
barrel, used for drowning, 19
Bartlett, Dr. Joseph, 72
base, 25
baths, 49
bateau, 68
battalion, 30
Battle of
    Bennington, 54
    Boston, 13, 41, 43
    Breed's Hill, 5, 13, 41
    Bunker Hill, 5, 13
    Charleston, 41
    Concord, 41, 65
    Guilford, 17
    Lexington, 41
    New York, 38, 43, 44, 48
    Princeton, 20, 56
    Saratoga, 41
    Yorktown, 41, 42
Baume, Colonel, camp stove, 54
bedding, camp, 52
bedding, shipboard, 61
belladonna, 23
benzoic acid, 12
Bethlehem, Pennsylvania,
    hospital, 44, 45
bifocals, 77
Bilious Plague, 15
bitten bullets, 38

"Bitter Apple," 23
Bladder in the throat, 14
Blane, Dr., on seaman's diseases, 56
blistering, 17
blistering iron, 64
blisters, 11, 12, 17
bloodroot, 20
blood-letting, 1, 8, 10, 12, 17
    bleeding bowl, 11
    chart, 11
    technique, 10
blue vitriol, 18
boats for wounded, 28
body fluids, 8, 9
body inversion, drowning, 19
bolsters, 30
borax, 24
borax symbol, 24
Boston, apprenticeship in, 2
Boston, military
    hospitals, 43, 46, 47
bottles, medicine, 22, 59
bottles, rum and liquor, 55
brace, knee, 34
Brazil root, 11
Breakbone Fever, 16
brimstone, 18
Bristol, Pennsylvania, hospital, 44
British Army medical systems, 5, 17
British hospitals, 43, 46, 47
British Light Infantry, 41
British occupation of Boston & British
    Seamen, 56
Brown, Dr. John, 9
Brown, Dr. William, 22
Brunonian System, 9
Burgoyne, General John, 57

C

calamina, 24
calomel, 12
Cambridge, Massachusetts, 43, 54
camp ailments, 13
    drowning, 19
    Heat Stroke, 18
    Impetigo, 18
    Infectious Arthritis, 17
    leg sores, 17
camphor, 12, 15, 25
campsites, 52
    air, 52
    bedding, 56
    heat, 52
    privies, 52, 53
    tenting, 52
camp stove, 54

Canada, Arnold's march to, 67–68
Cannibis Indica, 23
cannon ball wounds, 33
canteens
    bent wooden sides, 19
    iron strap, 19
    lathe-turned, 19
    wooden straps, 19
Capital Instruments
    amputation saw, 32
    amputation knives, 32
    crooked needle with ligature, 32
    probes, 32
    retractor, 32
    scalpel, 32
    screw tourniquet, 32
    tenaculum, 32
carts, 28
cartoons
    Dr. John Morgan, 5
    Dr. John Redman, 2
    satire on Rebel camps, 1
carboy, 21
cassia, extract of, 21
Carroll, Hermanus, dissection of, 2
castor oil, 12
cataplasms, 11, 17
cattarrh, 15
cathartics, 12,13
Certificate of Attendance, 3
chemist, 21
Chastellux, Marquis de, 27
Charleston, N.C., 58
Chester, John, 71
Chovet, Dr. Abraham, 3, 21
Church, Dr. Benjamin, 69
cigars, 15
cinnamon, 13
cloves, 13
clothing, cleanliness, 18
clysters, 11, 12, 13, 17
Cochran, Dr. John, 7
Cold Water Disease, 18
colds & causes, 15
    symptoms, 15
Colocynth, 23
Colonial militia, 1
Colonial legislature, 1
combs, American and British, 50
commissions, medical, 1
compresses, 27
Committee of Safety,
    Massachusetts, 65
    New Hampshire, 20
compound fractures, 36
Concord, Massachusetts, 1, 65
Congress
    Apothecary—General
        commissioned, 22

authorized Flying Camp, 36
discharge of Dr. Morgan, 7
increased pay scale, 64
medical regulations, 4
reorganization of Medical
        Department, 7
Connecticut Regimental buttons, 48
Connecticut requires examinations, 4
"contagions," 44
    Washington's, 54
Continental currency, 64
Continental Navy, 58
Continental pay, 48, 64
convalescent hospitals, 54
Cooke, Helena, 74
cooking pot, 54
Cornwallis, British General, 41
Corps of Invalids, 48
correctives, 25
Coste, Dr. Jean, 41, 42
counterirritants, 11
coward, 39
Cowpox Vaccine, 13
Craigie, Andrew, 74
crutch, 17
Cullen, Dr. William, 9
cups, *cowhorn*, 18
"Cyder-royal," 55
Cynanche Trachealis, 14

D
Dawes, William, 65–66
Deadly Nightshade, 23
Debility, treatment for, 9
Declaration of Independence, 49, 72
decoction, 25
Delaware River Crossing, 16
demulcents, 25
Dengue Fever
    causes, 16
    symptoms, 16
    illustration, 16
dentures
    Washington's first set, 40
    Washington's second set, 40
    lower dentures, 40
Devil's Bitt, 15
diaphoretics, 12
Diarrhea, 14
digestion, stage of, 31
dill, 13
dilating wounds, 33
Diphtheria
    causes, 14
    symptoms, 14
Director-General
    duty changes, 7
    problems faced by, 5, 6, 7
Director-Generals

Church, Dr. Benjamin, 5
Cochran, Dr. John, 7
Morgan, Dr. John, 5
Shippen, Dr. William, 7
dissections, 2, 3
"Dr. Froth," 49
"Doctor's Boy," 1
Dover's Powder, 12
Dragon's Blood, 23
dress, proper, 50
    hunting shirt, 50, 51
    soldier's rifle shirt, 51
    dropsy, 12
drowning & causes, 19
    treatments, 19
drug jar, 21
druggists, 21
    Trade marks, 21
dura mater, 37
Dysentery, 41, 44, 46
    causes, 14
    treatment, 14
Dyspepsia, 40

E
East Indian tree gum, 72
edema, 12, 14
Edinburgh, medical schools of, 1
elixir, 26
emetics, 12, 14
emollient, 26
Epidemical Eruptive Military Fever, 14
epidemics
    Colds, 15
    Dengue Fever, 16
    Diphtheria, 14
    Dysentery, 14
    Influenza, 15
    Malaria, 16
    Scarlet Fever, 15
    Smallpox, 13
    Tory-Rot, 16
    Typhoid, 14
    Typhus, 14
    Venereal Diseases, 16
    Yellow Fever, 15
Epilepsy, 40
Epsom Salt soaks, 11, 12
ergot, 23
European medicinals, 20
exciting causes of illnesses, 10
    removing irritability, 10
        blisters, 11
        blood-letting, 10
        cataplasms, 11
        clysters, 11
        formentation, 11
extracting active ingredients, 25
    decoction, 25

infusion, 25
tincture, 25
eyeglasses, 77
eye stone, 4

F
febrifuges, 12
ferns, 21
fever bark, 73
First South Carolina Line, 50
fish, 61
Fisher, Dr. Joshua, medical chest, 29
Fishkill, N.Y., hospital, 44
flaxseed, 11
fleams, 10
    Thomas Jefferson's, 10
    varieties of, 10
flour of sulphur, 25
Flux, 14, 52
Flying Camp, 7
Flying Hospital, 38
food preservation, 61
forceps, 31, 34
formentations, 11, 17, 26
Fort St. Frédéric, 40
foxglove, 73
fractures
    elbow, 35
    forearm, 35
    knee cap, 35
    lower leg, 35
    thigh, 35
Franklin, Ben, 72, 77
    Experiments in Electricity, 75
French Expeditionary Forces, 41
    hospital care, 41, 42
    introduce scalping, 40
    soldiers, 42

G
Gage, Thomas, 69
Galileo, observed temperature,
    pulse, 9
Galvani, Luigi, 75
Gardiner, Isaac, 65
garlic, 15
gas generating apparatus, 26
Gates, General Horatio, 57
Germantown, Pennsylvania
    wounded, 44
ginger, 13, 25
    symbol for, 24
glassware, 57
Glauber's Salts, 12
glycerine, 25
Great Sickness, 15
Greeks, ancient medicine of, 9
Greg, Captain, scalped, 39, 40
Guilford, North Carolina,

battle of, 17
gunpowder cleansing, 15
gunshot wounds, 34
gyrating chair, Rush's, 76

H
hair, 50
Hall, Dr. Lyman, 72
Hancock, John, 66, 69, 72
hard tack, 61
Harvard medical lectures, 3
healing principles, 30
heat, in camp, 52
Heat Stroke
    causes, 18
    symptoms, 18
    treatment, 18
hellebore, 23
hemlock, 25
herbs, 20
Hessians, 16, *41*, 68
Hippocrates, writings of, 1
"History of New York," Smith's, 4
hog's lard ointment, 18, 25
homesickness, 56
Homer, 27
honey, 25
    symbol, 25
honing stone, 30
Hooton, Elizabeth, 71
horehound, 13
horseradish, 13
hospital discipline, 48
hospital, Dr. Tilton's, 46
hospital tents, *47*, 48
hospital, log, 46
    plan, 46
Hospital, Continental Army
    duties, 4
    instrument scarcity, 30
    problems, 5, 6
    Regimental Surgeons, 6
    regulations, 5, 6
    reorganization by Congress, 7
    sanitation and crowding, 7
    staff, 4
    supplies, 5, 6
Hospital, Flying, 38
hospitals, 41, 42, 43, 44, 45
hospitals, American locations, 44
humors, 8
hunting shirts, 50, 51
Huntington, Ebenezer, 69
hygiene, personal
    hair, 50
    proper dress, 50
    shaving, 49
    shoes, 51
    skin, 49

I
Impetigo
    causes, 18
    symptoms, 18
    treatment, 18
Independence Day celebration, 6
Indian Hemp, 23
    herbs, 20
    Poke, 23
    shoes, 51
    sweat baths, 12
inflammation, stage of, 31
infusion, 25
inoculations, smallpox, 13
Infectious Arthritis
    causes, 17
    symptoms, 17
    treatment, 17
Intermitting Fever, 16
invasion of New Jersey, 38
Ipecac, 11, 12, 72
Ipecacuanha, 23
"Itch, the," 18

J
Jail Fever, 14
Jalap, 12
    root, 23
Jar, ointment, 21
jaundice, 15
Jones, Dr. John, 30, 49, 69
    clothing recommended, 51
    on quacks, 31
    privies, 52, 53

K
kettle, iron, 54
King petitioned, 57
Kings Bridge, N.Y. hospital, 48
King George, 77
Knox, General Henry, 68

L
lacerations, 33
Lancaster, Pennsylvania, 44
lantern, Old North Church, 65
"laudable pus," 31
laudanum, 12, 19
lavender, 13, 25, 72
Leg Sores, 17
licorice, 12
    root, 25
ligatures, 27, *33*
lime water, 18
"Limey," 60
Lind, Dr. James, 60, 73
lint, 62
liquor case, Washington's, 55
Long Island invasion, 6, 44, 48

London medical schools, 1
louse, *14*, 15
Lyonet, Pierre, microscope made by, 8

M
Macaon, ancient physician, 27
maggots, 38
magnesium sulfate, 12
Malaria
 causes, 16
 symptoms, 16
 treatment, 16, 73
Malignant Bilious Fever, 14
Manheim, Pennsylvania hospital, 44
marjoram, 13
Marshall, Christopher, Apothecary, 22
Massachusetts physical examinations, 4
mattresses, 52
Medical commissions, 1
 degrees, rarity of, 1
 Quack, 4
 standards, 1, 4
medical schools
 admissions requirements, 1
 colonial, 1
 curriculum, 1
 degree, 1
 European, 1
medications, 11
 antiarthritics, 11
 anodynes, 11
 antidysentery, 11
 antipyretics, 12
 diuretics, 12
 emetics, 12
 muscular spasm, 12
 purgatives (cathartics), 12
 sudorifics or diaphoretics, 12
medicinal roots, 20
medicinals, crude
 belladonna, 23
 Bitter Apple, 23
 ergot, 23
 Dragon's Blood, 23
 hellebore, 23
 Indian Hemp, 23
 jalap root, 23
 Ipecacuanha, 23
 Quaker button, 23
 Prickly Ash bark, 23
 rosemary, 23
 senna, 23
 tragacanth, 23
 wintergreen, 23
 vanilla bean, 23
medicine bottles, 22
 clay, 12
 glass, 12
medicine by numbers, 59

Medicine chest
 Dr. Joshua Fisher's, 29
 Dr. Benjamin Rush's, 16
 sea, 63
medicine dropper, 61
medicine, European
 British, 41
 French, 41
 German, 41
medicine jar, Delft, 22
medicine, lack of, 20
mental health, 76–77
Mercer, Dr. Hugh, 20, 38
 apothecary pill tile, 26
 apothecary shop, 20
 his bleeding bowl, 11
mercurial purgatives, 14
mercury, 12
 symbol, 24
methyl salicylate, 23
microdissection microscope, 8
Middle Department, Army, 49
"Military Journal," Thacher's, 4
militia, 48, 56, 57
 in Flying Camp, 38
 training and equipment, 1
 surrounding Boston, 4
milk, 16
mints, 25
mixture, 26
"mockasins," 51
Moore, Solomon, *shaving set*, 49
Moravians, Pennsylvania, 44, 45
Morgan, Director-General John, 2, 22
 character, 5
 Director-General problems, 5, 6
 discharged from duties, 7
 Hospital management, 43
 instruments for regiments, 29
 portrait of, 6
 surgical regulations, 27, 28, 29
Morristown, New Jersey, camp, 44
mortar and pestle
 brass, 25
 General Knox's, 24
mosquitoes, 15, 16, 17
mug, wooden, 18
Mulliken, Lydia, 66, 67
musket barrel for gases, 26
myrrh, 25

N
Naval Regulations, 61
needles, 62
nerve-muscle experiment, 8
nerve stimulation, 13
Newburyport, Massachusetts, broadside, 57
New England soldier, 56
New Haven, Connecticut, hospitals, 48

Newport, Rhode Island, 41
New York City, 43
 apprenticeship in, 2
 invasion of, 38, 43, 44, 48
 "Resurrectionists," 2
noggin, burl, 18
"Nostalgia," 56
nutmeg, 13
nux vomica, 23

O
oak bark, 18
oil of anise, 12, 72
ointments, 18, 33
opium, 11, 12, 31, 42
Orchid roots, Near East, 72

P
palace at Williamsburg, 43
Papoosquash Point, Rhode Island, 41
paregoric, 12
Parsons, Dr. Usher, 59
paste, 11
patriotic woman broadside, 57
patriotism, 1
Peekskill, New York, hospital, 44
Pennsylvania Hospital, 2
 apprentice system, 2
 awards, 2
 drawing of, 2
 Flying Camps, 7
Pennsylvania Moravians, 44
pepper, 13
Perkins, Dr. Elisha, 75
Peruvian Bark, 11, 18
Pharmacopoeia, 42
 America's first, 22
Philadelphia, Corps of Invalids, 48
Philadelphia, epidemic of 1762, 15
Philadelphia *Gazette*, 2
Philadelphia, inoculation in, 13
Philadelphia Medical College, 1, 2, 5, 7, 22
Physicians, Colonial, 1
 number practicing in 1775, 1
 (see also Regimental Surgeons)
pill box, wooden, 12
pill tile, 26
pistol, Scottish Flintlock, 66
pitching tents, 52
Plasmodium parasites, 16
plasters, 11, 17
pledgets, *36*, 62
Pleurisy
 symptoms, 58
 treatment, 58
Plummer's Pills, 12
Pneumonitis, 15, 44
poke weed, 21
porphyria, 77

poultices, *17*, 31, 34
potatoes, dried, 60
potassium carbonate, 12
preparing compounds
    additives, 25
    base, 25
    correctives, 25
    vehicles, 25
Prescott, Dr. Abel, 67
Prescott, Dr. Abel, Jr., 67
Prescott, Dr. Benjamin, 67
Prescott, Dr. Samuel, 66, 67
prescription, the first, 21
prevention of illness, 49
prickly ash bark, 23
prickly pear, 21
Princeton, Battle of, 56
privateers, 58
probes, 32, 34
"Protection Fever," 58
Providence, Rhode Island, 41
provisions, 53, 54
Pulmonary Consumption, 56
punctures, 33
purgatives, 12
Purple Heart, 39
"putrid effula," 53

Q
quacks, medical, 4
quinine, 11, 16

R
Randolph, Peyton, 57
"Random, Roderick" by Smollett, 61
razor, 49
    camp barber's, 30
rations, 54
Reading, Pennsylvania, hospital, 44
rectal medications, 11
Redman, Dr. John, 2
    cartoon of, 2
Regimental Surgeons, 1, 20
    examination of, 4
    hospital regulations, 5, 6
    instruments listed, 29
    lack of cooperation, 6
    surgical rules, 28, 29
regulations, surgical, 27, 28
"Resurrectionists," 2
    objections to, 3
retractor, 32, 37
retreat, 53
    from New York, 43
Revere, Paul, 65, 69
    engravings, 3, 8, 65
    border design, 70
Rheumatism, 17, 40
rhubarb, 12

Rickettsia, 14
rifle shirts, 50, 51
Rochambeau, French General, 41
rubefacients, 13
rosemary, 23
Rush, Dr. Benjamin, 1, 2, 15, 72, 76
    bloodletting, 10, 76
    evils of rum, 55
    decayed teeth, 40
    hospital description, 44, 46, 47
    hygiene, 50, 53
    "Medical Inquiries and
        Observations," 56, 57
    medicine chest, 16
    notes on Dr. Morgan, 7
    portrait, 13
    proper foods, 53
    shirts, hunting, 51

S
sage, 13
"Sailor Physician," 59
saline, 12
salivation, 12
saltpeter, 16
sanitation, hospital, 42
sarsaparilla, 21
sassafras, 21, 25
saw, amputation, 32
scales, medical, 69
scalp trophy, 40
scalpel, 32
scalping, 39
    technique, 39
scarcity, surgical instruments, 29, 30
Scarlet Fever, 14
screw tourniquet, 32
Scurvy, 41, 56
    symptoms, 60
    treatment, 60, 61, 73
Seasickness, 59, 60
Sea Surgeon, 58
sea surgery inventory, 61, 62
senna, 23
Senter, Dr. Isaac, 67
shaving, 49, 50
shaving set, 49
Shippen, Dr. William, 1, 38, 45, 49
    dissecting room, mob attack, 3
    Director-General, 7
    portrait, 7
    Professor of Anatomy, 7
    resignation, 7
    "scandalous practice," 7
    teacher, 2, 3
shoes, 51
sickbay, 61
simple wounds, 33
skin, care of, 49

sleds, 28
Smallpox, 14, 41
    inoculations, 13
    techniques, 13, 14
soap, 25
sovereign remedy, 21
spearmint, 13
sphygmomanometer, 9
spirits, 26
    rations, 55
    "Washington's off limits" order, 55
splints, 55, 62
    forearm, 35
    leg, 35
    thigh, 35
starch, 25
stethoscope, Laennec's, 9
    wooden, 9
Steuben, Baron von, 47
stimulants, 13
stimuli, 9, 10
stove, camp, 54
"Strangers Row," 45
stresses
    in battle, 56, 57
    on friend and enemy, 57
    on women, 57
stretcher, 28
Stuart, Gilbert, 40
sudorifics, 12
sugar, 25
    symbol, 24
sulphide of antimony, 24
sulphur, 18
    symbol, 24
    flowers of, 73
sumac roots, 16, 72
"sure specific," 21
surgeons, 1
surgery, 27
    minor, 1
    regulations, 27, 28, 29
surgical equipment, 29, 30
    instruments, 29
    scarcity, 29, 30
    scissors, 31
surgical quarters, 62
    after engagement, 63, 64
    preparation, 62, 63
    surgery during engagement, 63
surgery, frontier, 39
sutler, 55
sweat baths, 12
sweating, 8
Swieten, Baron van
    book on diseases, 49, 50
Sydenham, Dr. Thomas, 8, 9
Symbols
    one ounce, 25

one pinch, 25
one pint, 25
one pound, 25
powder, 26
to mix, 26
to pulverize, 25
to solve, 25
to take, 25
syrup jar, Delft, 22

T
tartar emetic, 12, 18
tax stamps, 67
teeth extraction, 40
temperature and stress, 56
tenaculum, 32, 36
tendon wounds, 34
tenting, 52
Thacher, Dr. James
    contamination from crowding, 38
    medical examination, his, 4
    on scalping, 39
theories, medical, 8, 9, 10
Thomas, Dr. John
    scissors and forceps, 31
Throat Distemper, 14
Thornton, Dr. Matthew, 72
thunder jug, 44
thyme, 25
Ticonderoga, New York, 57, 67
Tilton, Dr. James
    hospital changes, 41, 42
    hospital tents, 47
    military hospital book, 46
    portrait, 45
tincture, 25
tissue irritability, 13
    anodynes, 13
    cathartics, 13
    diet, 13
    rubefacients, 13
    stimulants, 13
tobacco, 15
toilet set, Washington's 53
tomahawk, 39
tombstone, Captain Moore's, 16
tongue scraper, 53
tooth extractor, 40
tooth-pulling, 1
toothache, 40
toothbrush, Washington's, 53
Tory, 58
Tory-Rot, 16
tourniquets, 27, 36, 62
tractors, Perkins, 75

tragacanth, 23
"Travels Through North America," 27
"Travels Through Life" by Dr. Rush, 13
Traitor, Dr. Benjamin Church, 5
tranquilizing chair, Rush's, 76
"Treatise of the Scurvy," 60
Trenton, New Jersey, attack on, 16
Trenton-Princeton Battle, 56, 68
trepanning, 37
trepine, 37, 38
tub bath, 18
tuberculosis treatment, 24
turpentine, 16, 25
Tussis Epidemica, 15
tweezers, 12
Typhoid
    causes, 14
    symptoms, 14
Typhus, 44, 45
    causes, 14
    symptoms, 14
    treatment, 14

U
Ulcerations, 17

V
vanilla bean, 23
vehicles
    demulcents, 26
    electuaries, 25
    elixir, 26
    emollient, 26
    formentation, 26
    liniments, 25
    mixture, 26
    ointments, 25
    pills, 25
    salves, 25
    spirits, 26
Venereal Diseases
    causes, 16
    treatment, 16
verdigris, 24
    symbol, 24
victuals, 53
    preservation of, 61
vinegar, 15
    symbol, 24
Virginia Convention, 43
Vitamin C, 73

W
wagons, 28
Waldo, Dr. Albigence, 74

Warren, Dr. John, 3, 41, 71–72
Warren, Dr. Joseph, 71
Warren, Mercy, 13
Washington, General George
    death of, 10, 14
    dentures, 40
    hospital reports, 48
    inoculation order, 13
    liquor case, 55
    medical organization, 4
    on Regimental Surgeons, 6
    Purple Heart order, 39
    retreat, 53
    reviewing troops, 6
    soldier's dress, 50
    toilet set, 53
    Trenton-Princeton Battles, 68
water, 54
"water carriages," 28
wax anatomical mold, 3
West Indies medicinals, 20
wheel-barrow, 28
Wigglesworth, Col. Samuel, 20
wigwam, Indian, 44
    construction of, 45
Williamsburg, Virginia, palace, 43
wine spirit symbol, 24
wintergreen, 21, 23
Winthrop, Hannah, 13
Withering, Dr. William, 73
wounds, 33
    bleeding, 34
    burns, 34
    cannon ball wounds, 34
    dressing of, 1
    gunshot wounds, 34
    punctures, 33
    simple, 32
    tendon wounds, 34

X
xanthoxyllum, 23

Y
Yellow Fever, 15, 16
    causes, 15
    symptoms, 15
    treatment, 15
Yorktown, Virginia, 14

Z
zinc acetate, 24